Better with Age

The Ultimate Guide to Brain Training

works by phyllis strupp

The Richest of Fare: Seeking Spiritual Security in the Sonoran Desert, Sonoran Cross Press, 2004. An exploration of the question posed by Albert Einstein: "Is the universe a friendly place?" Winner of the Independent Publisher award for Best Mind-Body-Spirit Book for 2005.

"Permanent Wealth: You CAN Take It with You!" in *All Shall Be Well: An Approach to Wellness,* edited by William S. Craddock Jr., Church Publishing, 2009. Tips on integrating personal finances into a generative way of life.

Faith and Nature: The Divine Adventure of Life on Earth, Church Publishing, 2010. A small-group, multigenerational engagement curriculum based on *The Richest of Fare.*

"Brain Wealth: Building a Fully Invested Brain" in *Fitness, Spa and Wellness in the Private Club*, Club Managers Association of America, 2013.

At Home in the Desert, Sonoran Cross Press, 2014. A one-act play for tweens. The story features the adventures of twelve-year-old Chloe, who learns valuable life lessons about love, loss, and bullying from Alex, a teen with autism, and from mysterious friends she encounters while lost in the Sonoran Desert.

www.phyllisstrupp.info

Better with Age

The Ultimate Guide to Brain Training

Phyllis Strupp, MBA
Brain Coach

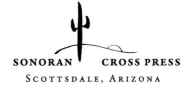

SONORAN CROSS PRESS
SCOTTSDALE, ARIZONA

Sonoran Cross Press LLC
8912 East Pinnacle Peak Road, Suite 604
Scottsdale, Arizona 85255

ISBN 978-0-9746727-1-7

Library of Congress Control Number: 2015913158

This book is not intended to offer medical advice, nor does it take the place of medical advice from a trained medical professional. Readers are advised to consult a physician or other qualified health professional regarding treatment of their specific medical problems. Neither the publisher nor the author assumes any responsibility for the consequences of any action taken by anyone following the information in this book.

Design and composition by Barbara Haines. The text is set in Calluna, the display in Affect and Whitney. The paper stock is 80 lb. white opaque smooth. Produced by Princeton Editorial Associates Inc., Scottsdale, Arizona. Printed by Bookmobile, Minneapolis, Minnesota.

9 8 7 6 5 4 3 2

For Mother Nature

CONTENTS

warning to the Reader

Dear Reader,
   If you are not interested in having a brain and a life that improve with age, don't bother reading *Better with Age: The Ultimate Guide to Brain Training,* as it will probably annoy you and waste your time and money.

   This book is also not suitable for the reader who meets one or more of the criteria below:

❋ Requires assurance that something is easy before taking it on

❋ Expects medical advice for a health problem

❋ Is unrepentantly irresponsible with time, words, emotions, or other potent substances

❋ Is convinced that wisdom from business, nature, science, or religion is useless

❋ Fears change and the word *transformation*

❋ Is unhappy to be alive

If you are ready to take charge of your brain assets and help them become better with age, then read on. This book is a suitable investment of time and effort for you.

Frequently Asked Questions

what is brain training?

The process by which someone deliberately exercises a brain area to develop a desired capability, skill, or mental range of motion.

will it hurt? No.

is it hard?

That depends on how motivated you are to accomplish your goal.

why should I bother?

To become a more complete and amazing human being.

how much time does it take? At least fifteen minutes a day.

how much does it cost?

The cost of this book and a big wad of self-curiosity.

does my age matter?

Yes. For best results, brain training must be tailored to fit a person's age, because the human brain has different strengths at different ages.

does it matter where I live?

Yes. The most significant influence on our brain is love, followed closely by culture, and people in different places have different ways of loving and living.

has the Better with Age approach to brain training worked for other people?

Yes. Hundreds of people between the ages of 10 and 100 have gotten results and increased their brain wealth with the *Better with Age* approach.

HOW old is the author? She was born in 1958.

HOW long has the author deliberately engaged the *Better with Age* approach to brain training? Since 2005.

HAS the *Better with Age* approach to brain training worked for the author?

You are in a better position to answer this question than the author.

A Note from the Author

Dear Reader,
I wish I could know more about you and what you are hoping to get out of this book. Perhaps you are looking for some new ways to follow the brain health advice to "use it or lose it." Or maybe you hope this book can be helpful to someone you know who is unfairly afflicted with one of the brain-related disorders that have become a household name these days, such as Alzheimer's, amyotrophic lateral sclerosis (ALS), anxiety, attention deficit hyperactivity disorder (ADHD), autism, bipolar disorder, dementia, depression, mild cognitive impairment (MCI), multiple sclerosis (MS), obsessive-compulsive disorder, Parkinson's disease, pervasive developmental disorder, post-traumatic stress disorder, psychosis, schizophrenia, or traumatic brain injury.

Alas, you and your motives for reading this book will remain a mystery to me. In a way, it doesn't really matter, because your brain knows what you need from this book, and will point you in the right direction as you read along.

I hope you will find what you are looking for in *Better with Age*, and along the way forge a whole new relationship with your brain—or as you will find I like to call it, *our brain*. But since I will be your guide on the learning adventure that lies ahead, and you may not have met a brain coach before, it's only fair that you know a little more about me and my qualifications to lead the way.

First and foremost, I am just as strange as everyone else, and perhaps even a little more so. I acquired a most peculiar habit when I was four years old, when my family lived in Escondido, California. One afternoon, I was in my bedroom with our cat, Whitey. He was lying on the bed,

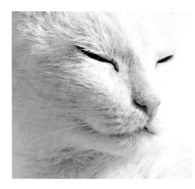

trying to nap. I put my ear on the soft white fur of his stomach. He didn't squirm or run off, so I closed my eyes to listen to his purr.

The resonant sound made me tingle from head to toe and float away from the "real" world. I had never experienced anything so glorious! After a bit, I got up and saw that the pressure of my head was making Whitey drool on the bedspread. I was horrified that I might have hurt him while in my blissful state, but Whitey was a tough old tomcat, and all was well.

Ever since then, I have been drawn to the invisible, "purr" side of life, while most other people seem to prefer the visible, "fur" side. What the ancient Celts called the "unseen worlds" seem more real to me than to most people. This trait has proved to be particularly useful in pursuing my vocation as a hopemonger, first in finance and then in brain coaching.

Better with Age is the product of a bomb that went off in my mind long ago, on a steamy summer night in New York City. Just after my graduation from Columbia Business School in May 1982, I began a financial management trainee job at the Dun & Bradstreet Corporation's headquarters on Park Avenue. As a freshly minted twenty-four-year-old MBA with student loans, I lived in an illegally sublet, Upper East Side apartment on a high floor with no air conditioning. On muggy evenings, I looked for ways to spend time in air-conditioned buildings after work without spending any money.

Back then, the museums in New York City stayed open late on Thursdays, with free public admission. That summer, I visited a different museum every Thursday evening and stayed until they kicked me out. During my visit to the American Museum of Natural History, I came upon an exhibit in a remote corner of the cool basement that consisted of a line of goofy-looking, life-sized models of human ancestors going back millions of years. A sign in front of a hairy modern human playing a wooden flute indicated that humans had been making music for about forty thousand years.

All of a sudden, my mind seemed to explode, and the questions flew like shrapnel. What made our ancestors wake up one day and start to make music? What did their music sound like? How did they figure out how to do it? What else might we wake up and do one day that we have never done before? What might *I* wake up and do one day that I have never done before? I was staring at the exhibit, lost in thought, when a security guard came around to throw me out.

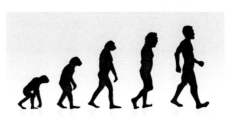

"Go back! It's a trap!"

Once I got back to my sweat lodge of an apartment, questions about the origins of music quickly receded behind the more immediate concerns of daily living. Little did I know that this was the first hint of a calling that would lead me to *Better with Age*.

A few years later, I met and married my soul mate, Peter, and we moved to Princeton, New Jersey. I became a financial services representative in February 1988, and a couple of years later Peter started his own publishing services business. We both became hard-working, self-employed professionals in hot pursuit of meaningful achievement and, of course, MORE MONEY. We assumed that happiness would follow our career and financial success.

In my job as a financial representative, my days were filled with the challenges of turning clients' financial worries into a plan of action to get MORE MONEY and be happy. But as the years went by, I noticed that, contrary to everyone's expectations, MORE MONEY did not seem to make anyone any happier or healthier. The statistics of my work were backing up this impression: the leading causes of white-collar disability insurance claims were nervous and mental conditions such as depression.

I wondered if there was something more important in life than MORE MONEY. Was it having children? We had opted not to have children, but having kids did not seem to relieve others of their concerns about MORE MONEY.

A move to Arizona in 1997 provided new horizons, literally and figuratively. Our mission statement for the move was "More time together outdoors." This new lifestyle introduced a change in my mental landscape as well. I began thinking about what might matter more in life than get-

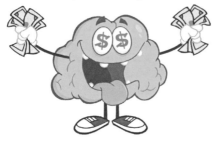

ting MORE MONEY. Returning to the questions that had arisen on that hot, steamy summer night at the museum in New York some twenty years before, I began to consider some new ones as well.

Reading *Walden* by Henry David Thoreau changed my view of nature and how I fit into it. Participating in a spiritual formation program for laity called Education for Ministry introduced me to the Bible and theology and reawakened my interest in history, my major in college.

My soul searching for what matters more than MORE MONEY was eventually framed by what Albert Einstein described as the most important question one can ask oneself: Is the universe a friendly place? My attempts to answer this question generated my first book, *The Richest of Fare: Seeking Spiritual Security in the Sonoran Desert,* published in 2004.

One line in *The Richest of Fare* summarizes my answer to Albert's question: "It's the relationships, stupid." Just like elementary particles of the universe, we are defined by our relationships. The meaningful connections we build with other people, nature, the divine, and our own selves make the universe a friendly place. Our relationships matter more than MORE MONEY.

While writing *The Richest of Fare,* I became aware that the brain—our gateway to consciousness—was the most valuable asset we humans own. One line I wrote pointed the way to my future career as a brain coach: "Cerebral wealth, not financial wealth, is the key to over-coming fear and having faith in a

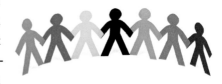

friendly higher power." But it took me until 2007 to make that next step.

In 2005, I was selected to serve on the faculty of CREDO, the Episcopal Church's clergy wellness program. Guided by a faculty team, the eight-day CREDO conferences allowed participants to focus on personal issues related to health, finances, vocation, spirituality, and human relationships in the context of identity and a relationship with God. My task was to help attendees review their finances.

Before this, I had met very few clerics. I wondered whether the clergy would be any different in their attitude toward their finances than the dentists, doctors, lawyers, executives, and small business owners I had worked with for twenty years. Surely, I thought, they would be more spiritually prepared to deal with the demon of MORE MONEY.

Teaching at some twenty-six conferences in six years, I met more than six hundred members of the clergy, working one on one with most of them. I came to the conclusion that clerics were different from my previous clients with regard to finances in two ways. First, they made the same mistakes as everyone else, but they felt ten times worse about them. Second, they were so attracted to mystery that they tolerated mystery in strange places, such as their checking accounts and net-worth statements. As a group, these clerics were no more spiritual about money than anyone else—maybe even less so. But the few who did have a well-formed spiritual attitude toward money taught me what mind-body-spirit generativity looks like in daily life.

Teaching for CREDO exposed me to a wide range of professionals and research about mental and physical health, furthering my understanding of the human experience from a mind-body-spirit perspective. I could see how my understanding about the brain could be applied to real-life problems. In 2007, I quit my day job in financial services to pursue a career as a brain coach.

In 2009, I graduated from the Brain Research in Education certificate program offered by the University of Washington–Seattle. The purpose of this program was to teach participants how to educate the public about the research findings of cognitive neuroscience (linking brain activity with behavior) in a responsible, ethical manner.

This program and subsequent conferences for educators triggered a huge paradigm shift in my thinking about the brain. Until this point, I had been under the delusion that my brain was *my* most valuable asset— it belonged to *me*, like the rest of my body. After the shift, I began to

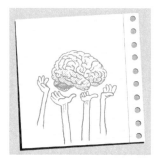

realize that my brain was a *social organ*. My brain tissue was being sculpted by relationships with my fellow human beings, whether I liked it or not. My brain was really *our brain*. Once again, I was confronted by the message "It's the relationships, stupid."

There's a reason why the Oracle of Delphi said "Know thyself" rather than "Rely on thyself." Our brains are highly vulnerable to fear, stress, and health problems when we try to do too much alone. Like all other virtues, self-reliance has to be contained to avoid becoming a vice. But we're getting ahead of ourselves—more on this later.

As I continued my work as a brain coach, it dawned on me that the financial world had a few tricks up its sleeve that could be useful for brain training. Our 100 billion neurons are valuable to us. Why not manage our cerebral treasure with some of the same effective techniques we employ to manage our financial wealth, such as asset allocation and portfolio management? Thus were born the learning devices of brain assets and the Brain Portfolio Tool, which you'll learn more about in chapters 3 and 4.

Over the years, I have had the privilege to work with a wide variety of people from ages 10 to 100. The contents of this book are the product of seven years of experimentation by these willing pioneers, who have improved their brain performance using my approach and asked me to put it in writing. The poster child for the *Better with Age* approach is my husband, Peter. You'll hear more about his inspiring story in the pages ahead.

I am deeply grateful to all the family, friends, colleagues, and clients who have helped *Better with Age* come to life, both in and beyond the pages of this book. I would also like to thank the talented team of professionals that used their diverse talents to produce this book, including Laurel Muller (art), Barbara Haines (design and composition), Peter Strupp (everything), and especially my editor Erika Büky, whose "reader empathy" and breadth and depth of insight are astounding.

Better with Age provides the tools to take charge of our cerebral assets and put them to work so that both our brains and our lives improve with age. We'll explore a whole new approach to "Use it or lose it" that moves way beyond crossword puzzles, Sudoku, or computer games. These activities don't challenge the parts of the brain that need the most exercise to get better with age.

The intended audience for this book is individuals of any age, but especially forty and over, who are more interested in practice than theory with regard to brain training. Tools, tips, techniques, and real-life stories are provided throughout the book. Terms that are included in the glossary appear in bold italics. Additional resources, including a few references, are provided at the end of the book. The resources are organized by both chapter and type (publications, research articles and studies, and websites).

At the end of each chapter, engagement questions are provided to facilitate personal reflection and small-group discussions. Ideally, I'd like to see *Better with Age* investment clubs springing up like dandelions all over the world, discussing ways to get rich quick with brain wealth.

By the time you're done reading *Better with Age,* you will be in a powerful position to write your own brain-training success story and keep winning at the most important game of all: the game of life. *Human life. Your* human life.

So now, are you ready to embark on our learning adventure? All aboard!

Carefree, Arizona
July 4, 2015

Why spend your money on what is not bread,
and your labor on what does not satisfy?
Listen, listen to me, and eat what is good,
And your soul will delight in the richest of fare.

Isaiah 55:2

Introduction

> Be a Columbus to whole new continents and worlds within you, opening new channels, not of trade, but of thought. HENRY DAVID THOREAU, *Walden*

We are beginning a voyage of discovery that will be a wild goose chase unless an important fact is understood right up front. Fine wine is designed to improve with age—and so is the human brain. Over age 40, the rest of our body cannot get better with age, but our brain can, thanks to a magic trick called **neuroplasticity**. Neuroplasticity is a healthy brain's secret weapon for improving with age, and it is the primary focus of brain training.

Our brain's main business is conducted by highly specialized cells of the **nervous system** called **neurons,** also referred to as *"gray matter."* Neurons come in many different shapes and sizes and perform many different functions. They are very sociable little cells, spending their days chatting and working with other neurons. They are also very intelligent cells, capable of counting and providing each other with feedback such as "speak up, I can't hear you" or "tone it down."

But neurons insist on having their elbow room. They do not physically touch each other, because a little gap, called a **synapse,** separates each neuron from its next-door neighbors. Neurons communicate with each other by exchanging electrochemical messages across the synapse, like neighbors passing notes through a hole in a wall (see figure I.I).

A working relationship between two neurons is called a **synaptic connection**. Synaptic connections between neurons, also known as "white matter," underwrite all of our brain's activity. The more often neurons work together, the stronger the connections between them and the more efficient their teamwork. As the neuroscientists say, the neurons that fire together, wire together. However, too much or too little

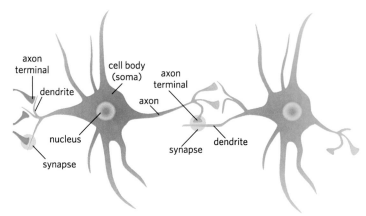

Figure I.1. Neurons communicate by exchanging chemical messages at the synapse.

interaction can make neurons unbalanced, producing a state of **neurosis** in an individual.

Each neuron can have thousands of synaptic connections with other neurons. The average adult has a three-pound brain that contains some 100 billion neurons and 500 trillion synaptic connections, with room for 500 trillion more connections in the same size skull. With all this connectivity, the human brain is reckoned to be the most complex structure in the known universe. In other words, we have inherited the best brains in the world!

Of course, there's a catch to having our superstar brain: it comes with some warranty conditions. Mother Nature has been tinkering with animal brains for 500 million years to invent a brain like ours. She has not entrusted us with these turbocharged brains to sit around performing mindless brain-training exercises on a computer, like caged hamsters on a wheel. She has great expectations for us! The most complex structure in the universe is designed for activities a whole lot more important and rewarding than games and puzzles.

Our brains are sitting around up there, awaiting our commands. Neurons will do the work we give them to do, as long as we keep bugging them to get the job done. But building new synaptic connections is a lot of work, so our thrifty brain only bothers to do this when it is really necessary.

When someone wants something with their whole heart, our brain can work miracles to comply, as the inspiring recovery of Gabrielle Giffords demonstrates.

Neuroplasticity in Action

On January 8, 2011, a troubled young man opened fire on a crowd in Tucson, Arizona, with a semi-automatic 9mm Glock pistol, wounding thirteen people and killing six. The target of this bloody attack was the forty-one-year-old U.S. Representative Gabrielle Giffords, who was shot at close range. A bullet entered the back of her head, tearing a tunnel through the left side of her brain.

Ms. Giffords was in surgery at Tucson's University Medical Center within thirty-eight minutes of the shooting. Her doctors announced that if the bullet had followed a slightly different path or passed through the right side of her brain instead, she probably would not have survived. Based on their knowledge of the duties of the injured brain areas, they predicted that she would survive but was likely to face long-term difficulties with vision, language, speech, and movement on the right side of her body. These early predictions proved to be spot on.

The determined Ms. Giffords made a remarkable recovery, aided by excellent medical care, physical therapy, social support, her own hard work—and her brain's neuroplasticity. Her brain grew new connections to compensate for losses in the damaged areas. Even so, on the second anniversary of the tragedy, Ms. Giffords revealed in a news interview that she still had difficulty with vision on her right side, finding the right words to use, speaking, moving the toes on her right foot, and walking.

On the third anniversary, she shared this surprising update: "This past year, I have achieved something big that I've not spoken of until now. . . . Three years ago, I did not imagine my right arm would move again. For so many days, it did not. I did exercise after exercise, day after day, until it did. . . . It took a long time, but my arm moves when I tell it to."

The story of Gabrielle Giffords confirms that our brain can grow new synaptic connections to work around impaired or dead neurons *in response to persistent requests.* Enabling neuroplasticity in this way is the key not only to Ms. Giffords' successful outcome but also to the brain-training techniques in *Better with Age*. In later chapters we'll hear from individuals who have applied these techniques, with persistence and determination, to marshal neuroplasticity and succeed in a variety of personal quests.

There is no need to sit around waiting for a traumatic brain injury in order to follow Ms. Giffords' example. But for most people, the hardest part of brain training is figuring out what you want to do. What *you* want to do, not what others want you to do—and what you want to do with your whole heart.

The most mysterious aspect of all this is how we can take a third-party view of our brain. If you or I want something that our brains cannot currently do, we must be *something more* than our brain activity. What is the *something more*? Where does it come from? Where does it live inside of us? No one knows.

Fortunately, we do not need to solve these mysteries to succeed with brain training. However, we must engage our brain assets to access the full ***mental range of motion*** they provide. As the neuroscientists say, use it or lose it.

Making the most of our brain in this way enables each one of us—as well as the human species—to become better with age.

'Tis a lesson you should heed: Try, try, try again.
If at first you don't succeed, Try, try, try again.
WILLIAM EDWARD HICKSON

---

our Mental Range of Motion

The verb *train* means to cause someone or something to develop an ability, skill, or way of thinking with a particular objective in sight. Effective brain training is simply working our neurons in new ways to enable neuroplasticity to get something we really want. Lifelong learning *that is personally meaningful* is the key to brain health and neuroplasticity.

Training the brain is similar to training the rest of the body. Physical training aims to develop the body's capabilities for a desired outcome, be it athletic achievement, sex appeal, or vitality. The major dimensions of physical fitness include:

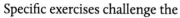

* Balance
* Endurance
* Flexibility
* Mobility
* Strength

Specific exercises challenge the body to improve in different ways. For example, weight training boosts the strength of muscles and bones, while stretching makes joints more limber, and aerobic exercise makes the heart pump more efficiently to build stamina. Challenging our bodies in all these ways maximizes our body's capabilities and helps us to stay active and healthy.

Brain training aims to make the most of the brain's capabilities for a desired outcome, be it career advancement, personal growth, improved relationships, self-esteem, inner peace, happiness, or healing, as in Gabrielle Giffords' case. As we will learn in chapter 3, each brain asset contributes a certain range of mental motion that helps build brain health and well-being. The mental dimensions of our brain assets include:

* Achievement
* Adaptation
* Adventure
* Attachment
* Autobiography

Specific activities also challenge our brain to improve its level of fitness and expand its capacities. The key difference between training the body and the brain lies in the type of activities that provide exercise. The body has to move to get exercise. However, the brain gets a workout through the exercise of the body, mind (thoughts), or spirit (feelings).

Physical exercise is good for our brain; but so are art, chess, meditation, singing, and writing, even though they don't involve much physical activity. The best forms of brain exercise work both the body and the

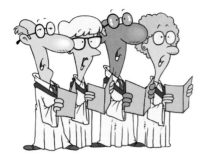

brain: for example, acting, dancing, or tai chi. In chapters 4 and 5, we'll delve into brain-training activities and techniques in more depth.

Our brain requires all three forms of exercise (of body, mind, and spirit) to flourish. Using our full range of mental motion maximizes our ability to get better with age as a *whole person*. We can maintain our vitality as we age by exercising mind and spirit to compensate for bodily decline and protect our brain from stress-related inflammation.

All movements expressed in body, mind, or spirit have a common source: emotion, from the Latin words "to move from."

Distinguishing Gain and Loss

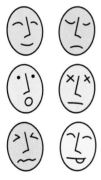

Emotions are the physiological sensations we feel of the universe within us. Every day, we experience the upbeats, the downbeats, the cacophonies, and the harmonies of the electrons and neutrinos, the neutrons and protons within the atoms that form our bodies. Where else could emotions come from? Whatever the answer may be, emotions have one major purpose: to help our brain distinguish between a gain and a loss, unencumbered by moral concerns.

No one wakes up in the morning and says, "I want to be a loser today." Our brains are always on the hunt for our next gain, big or small, to make us feel like a winner! Pursuing gains and avoiding losses is our brain's top priority. To fulfill this mission, our brain wields a very powerful tool: the stress-response system.

When the opportunity to score a gain (pleasure) or avoid a loss (pain) arises, an emotion is triggered. Biochemical signals guide our brain to respond adaptively, given our **personality**, memories, goals, perception, and values related to the current situation. To generate resources for quick action, our brain has a hotline to the body: the **hypothalamus**-pituitary-adrenal (HPA) axis. By quickly releasing the hormone **cortisol** into the bloodstream, the HPA axis activates the stress-response system, ordering the heart and lungs to work harder and the digestive and immune systems to slow down.

Let me give you an example of how our brain and body use this hotline to manage our stress-response system. One day, I was hiking with friends in the desert and looked down for a moment. Next to my foot I saw something round, still, and silent, the same color as the surrounding rock. Before I even knew what it was, I had hopped back quickly and screamed a warning to my hiking buddies, who also jumped away fast. It was a rattle-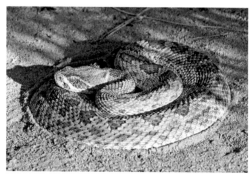snake, but it hadn't rattled a warning as we approached. Fortunately, no one (including the snake) was harmed by the encounter.

So once the mind signals that things around us have settled down, the brain flips the switch to settle things down within us: the *vagus nerve*, shown in figure 1.2. This cranial nerve connects the brain to the body's organs to deactivate the stress-response system and activate the relaxation response. The calming effects of the vagus nerve allow the brain and body to return to their happy place (*homeostasis*), the optimal state for enjoying good health. We can deliberately activate the vagus nerve's soothing activity *at any time* through deep breathing.

Every day, we experience a wide variety of "inner movements" (emotions) that help our brain make sense of the world *from our personal perspective*. When we perceive a threat, the stress-response system engages. If we do not adapt to the threat and relax, the vagus nerve does not tell the organs to relax.

Continuing engagement of the stress-response system carries a heavy cost. Cortisol, *norepinephrine,* and other stress hormones increase *inflammation* and can disrupt sleep. Over time, chronic inflammation can wreak havoc with *gut bacteria* that allow the absorption of nutrients from food and run the immune system. When gut bacteria are happy,

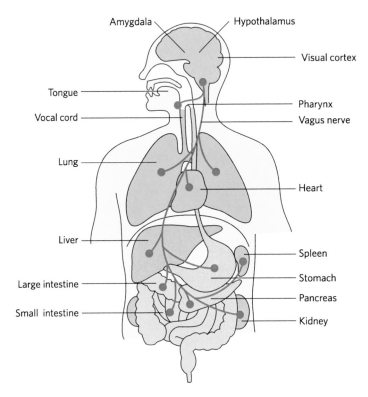

Amygdala · Hypothalamus

Visual cortex

Tongue

Pharynx

Vocal cord · Vagus nerve

Lung

Heart

Liver

Spleen

Large intestine · Stomach

Pancreas

Small intestine

Kidney

Figure I.2. The vagus nerve (shown in blue) disengages the stress-response system, allowing the body to relax.

the product of the gastrointestinal tract is log-shaped, like the colon itself. When gut bacteria are upset, constipation, diarrhea, or other irregular shapes occur.

Stress can also expedite aging and wear and tear on our *telomeres.* Healthy telomeres, the little caps at the end of our chromosomes that keep our genes from unraveling, are linked to living long and well.

Inflammation-related damage to telomeres and gut bacteria is the suspected link between toxic emotional activity and major diseases linked to stress, including Alzheimer's, arthritis, cancer, diabetes, and heart disease.

The brain cannot manage our powerful stress-response system alone. It is our responsibility to use the mind to calm the brain and body. In addition to deep breathing, the most potent weapon we have for stress management is verbal access to mental states—turning feelings into words so we can understand and manage them. When no imminent danger is present, we need to figure out how to cope with loss (real or perceived), and move on to our next gain.

Resilience—the ability to help the brain and body move quickly back to homeostasis—is an important life skill required for maintaining neuroplasticity and getting better with age. In chapters 6 and 7, we'll learn more about how to manage stress and master resilience.

Ultimately, our lifestyle must encourage neuroplasticity to help us get better with age. What good does it do us to train our brain for an hour and then work against it the rest of the day? Chapter 7 will introduce us to the Super-Agers, the most resilient people in the world, who can offer us some lifestyle tips for maintaining neuroplasticity to age 100 and beyond.

Brain fitness is not an end in itself but a means to the end of becoming a bigger, better, more resilient person who enjoys these advantages in life:

* Full range of mental motion
* Happy gut bacteria
* Healthy, long telomeres
* Integration of inner and outer lives
* Meaning and purpose in serving others
* Neuroplasticity
* Warm, intimate relationships

Our brain is after a Hollywood ending for our lives. Our unfolding life story should resemble a stock market chart: it should show ups and downs, trending up over time. To achieve this outcome, *perceived gains must offset perceived losses* over the long haul. We must navigate our gains and losses to keep feeling like a winner. Emotions and feelings must be kept in check to make sure the stress-response system is used mainly for major threats.

In the chapters ahead, we will continue our learning adventure to explore training our brain for the purpose of becoming better with age.

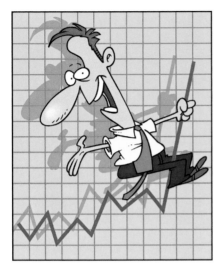

We will learn more about how our brain came to be as it is and how to manage our brain assets like a well-balanced portfolio to maximize our vitality returns.

Let's begin with the end in mind. Successful training of any type requires a vision of the desired outcome. What does it look like when we use all of our brain assets and full range of mental motion—attachment, achievement, adventure, adaptation, autobiography—to navigate the twists and turns of life well? At the next stop along our journey, we'll consider what successful brain training looks like amid the battle conditions of daily life.

> The highest stage in moral culture at which we can arrive is when we recognize that we ought to control our thoughts. . . . As Marcus Aurelius long ago said, "The soul is dyed by the thoughts."
> CHARLES DARWIN, *The Descent of Man*

Engagement questions

1. What are you hoping to learn from *Better with Age* and why?

2. What activities did you consider as brain exercise before reading this book?

3. What dimension of your mental range of motion would you like to widen at this time: achievement, adaptation, adventure, attachment, autobiography?

4. What feelings do you enjoy the most? What people, situations, or activities trigger these feelings for you?

5. What situations trigger stress for you? What techniques do you use to manage toxic emotions?

6. How well do you sleep at night? What disrupts and promotes good sleep for you?

7. Who do you know who has bounced back from a traumatic injury or major loss? What attitudes and behaviors aided their recovery?

8. How do you see your unfolding life story: trending up or trending down?

what success Looks Like

 Every man if he so desires becomes sculptor of his own brain.
Santiago Ramón y Cajal

We live in the best of times and the worst of times for having a brain. On the one hand, exciting research findings about neuroplasticity and aging have created a media buzz about our brain and how we can realize its vast potential.

On the other hand, skyrocketing rates of mental malfunction across all age groups in the United States have triggered widespread fear about becoming part of the neurological underclass. Consumers are susceptible to hype and promises of easy fixes. Good news, such as a dramatic reduction in the rate of Alzheimer's in the worst-hit countries (including the United States, Sweden, and Germany) doesn't always make the headlines or the Alzheimer's Association's home page.

The mass media is far better than the scientific community at turning research into news you can use, but reader beware. Brain hype that benefits advertisers and media companies more than consumers is widespread. Articles and TV news stories would have you believe that blueberries, computer games, crossword puzzles, physical exercise, advanced degrees, red wine, or expensive supplements made of rare berries from Tibet are all you need to avoid Alzheimer's, but this is not the case.

Brain researchers have yet to answer the basic questions, "What keeps the brain healthy?" and "What causes Alzheimer's?" Lifestyle and environmental factors affecting genetic expression drive some 95 percent of Alzheimer's cases, but the factors remain elusive. Well-educated people who run five miles a day and eat healthy foods can get Alzheimer's, while others with "unhealthy" habits may live long with excellent cognitive function until the end. Important factors such as stress, environmental toxins, culture, and sleep quality are difficult to quantify, and thus are often overlooked by researchers. No one knows the extent to which personal lifestyle choices determine who gets the disease and who does not. But neuroscientists agree on one thing when it comes to the brain: use it or lose it.

In the meantime, confusion abounds about how the brain works and what we can do to keep it healthy. I have encountered this brain bewilderment daily at work and sometimes even at home.

From Losing It to Using It

One spring morning in 2008, my husband, Peter, and I were out for a morning walk. Out of the blue, this healthy fifty-two-year-old man declared, "I think I'm losing it." Resisting the temptation to respond, "You finally noticed!" I asked why he thought this way.

He said that his mind was not as sharp as it used to be; he was taking longer to remember names and information. Furthermore, because his paternal grandmother, who had lived to be a hundred, had struggled with Alzheimer's for decades, he was convinced that he had the gene and that the process had already set in.

I shared with him the observation from a researcher at a conference that some 95 percent of Alzheimer's cases are not linked to the genes you are born with. This information was consistent with his own family's situation, as evidenced by the fact that his own father was aging quite well in his late eighties, even though his mother had had Alzheimer's. (Six years later, his father died suddenly at ninety-two while on vacation in Germany, cognitively fit as a fiddle.)

Peter was also unaware that over age forty, our brain deliberately slows down when retrieving information, searching more *memory* records for every task it performs, to facilitate integration and wisdom. What he saw as a sign of Alzheimer's was actually an indicator of normal brain function at fifty-two!

We discussed how our brain is built to get better with age, as long as it is challenged to do new, personally meaningful activities. He had been in the same kind of work for over thirty years, so I wondered out loud if his brain needed an exciting adventure outside of work, like a new hobby. He said, "Hmmmm."

At first, nothing changed. Peter continued in his same old lifestyle. But a few months later, a friend was looking for someone to play the role of the king in a children's play called *The Plastic Touch.* Peter had enjoyed acting in high school and was longing to return to it. Playing the king appealed to his ego, so he took the part.

Peter stopped talking about losing it and got busy using it. Acting tapped his brain assets differently than his computer-intensive, sedentary day job as an editor. At work, he was using his occipital lobe (visual activity), temporal lobe (language), and frontal lobe (planning, problem solving, project management) quite vigorously, especially on the left side.

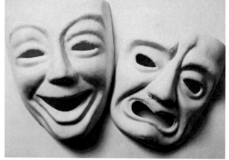

Acting required him to use the right side of his brain—from back to front—more strenuously. During many hours of rehearsal every week, he was learning new things, interacting with people, standing and moving, memorizing lines, and imagining how his character would feel, speak, and act.

Not surprisingly, Peter's brain rose to the challenge of this new workout. He was amazed at the way his brain could memorize lines which he could then recall effortlessly, the mental equivalent of developing automatic "muscle memory." There was no more talk about losing it or getting Alzheimer's.

Peter performed the role of the king quite well, and he enjoyed it, too. The director was quick to notice that he showed up on time, remembered his lines, and willingly followed her directions, so she gave him additional acting opportunities.

Within a year, he became involved with our local community theater. At first, he had told them he was only interested in acting—no singing or dancing. Over time, this theater group got him to sing and dance on stage in an ensemble. In 2011, he performed in two plays at

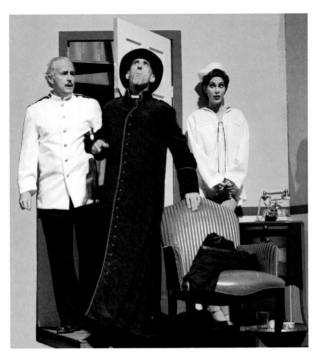

Figure 1.1. Peter Strupp (left) on stage as the Purser in *Anything Goes*, Desert Foothills Theater, November 2014.

the same time—taking a lead role in one—and his memory never failed him.

But the greatest test of his cognitive abilities came in the autumn of 2014, when a favorite director asked him to play the role of the Purser in the Cole Porter musical *Anything Goes*. He had to act, sing, and dance in many numbers to the strict standards of a choreographer who was a former Rockette!

He came back from the first few rehearsals totally demoralized. He even said to the director and choreographer, "Take me out of these numbers if I'm not good enough—I'm just not getting it." They said he was fine, and they'd let him know if he wasn't. I reassured him that it was taking his brain a little longer than usual to learn because his father had just died two months earlier.

He kept working at it, getting help from more adept members of the cast. He would practice in our living room, moving his hands around and saying things like "Neighbor, self, self, neighbor" to remember how he needed to move. To his own surprise, he and his brain were able to pull all this off. He looked great on stage in his uniform, as you can see in figure 1.1. Friends and family were amazed and impressed—including me.

These acting adventures occurred while Peter was working full time running his own business. This took a lot of energy, working all day and acting at night and on weekends. He was fueled by the vitality and joy that come from making the most of our brain assets in personally meaningful ways.

As an amateur actor, he did not earn any money, but he cashed in on brain wealth. His five brain assets built new connections that expanded his mental range of motion in all five categories: attachment, achievement, adventure, adaptation, and autobiography.

Now he expects his brain to improve with age, and it is doing just that. He looks ahead and thinks about retirement not as an escape from work but as an exciting, *generative* time of "rewirement."

Peter's story demonstrates an important truth. Our brain is like the rest of our body: it can get out of shape, and it can also get fit. But it's hard to buff up something you can't see or understand. In chapter 4, we will learn about the Brain Portfolio Tool, a framework to "see" our brain as a set of assets that need to be managed for long-term growth.

Whatever approach to brain training you use, the desired outcome is the same: to keep the brain fully invested as long as you live to get better with age.

Live Long and Prosper

Thanks largely to our high-powered brain, the human species has one of the longest life spans of any land mammal. But living long is not the same as living well, as we can see by comparing the life stories of two rich and famous twentieth-century contemporaries: Ronald Reagan and Pablo Picasso.

Born in Illinois in 1911, Ronald Reagan became the fortieth president of the United States in 1981 and lived to the ripe old age of ninety-three. He did everything one is supposed to do to avoid Alzheimer's, such as maintaining a healthy diet, physical exercise, social support, and engage-

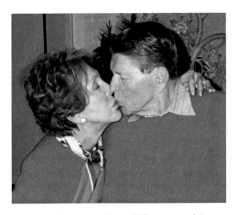

Figure 1.2. Nancy and Ronald Reagan on his 89th birthday in February, 2000.

ment in meaningful activities. Even so, he spent the last decades of his life struggling with cognitive decline. In 1994, he announced to the public he had Alzheimer's disease. Ten years later, he died, after a long goodbye.

In contrast to President Reagan, Pablo Picasso died at age ninety-one with his boots on, cognitively speaking. Picasso was born in Málaga, Spain, in 1881 and went on to become one of the most influential artists of the twentieth century. In 1973, he died suddenly while he and his wife Jacqueline entertained friends for dinner at home in Mougins, France.

A secret room discovered after his death revealed that Picasso had also been one of the twentieth century's great sculptors, yet few had known it. He had spent the last decades of his life creating beautiful sculptures that could have sold at high prices but instead were kept for his private collection.

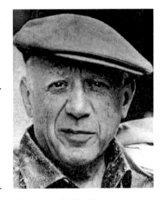

Figure 1.3. Pablo Picasso at age 80.

Reagan managed to live a long time, but Picasso managed to *live long and prosper* —as Mr. Spock used to say on *Star Trek*— and end his life story on a high note. This is not to say that either one of these men got what they deserved. No one can explain why some people get Alzheimer's. Many different factors can trigger dementia-like symptoms, including head injuries, heavy metals, industrial chemicals, mold, neurotoxins in plants, parasites, and who knows what else. But what can be safely said is that all of these assaults rob our brain of its highest abilities—our "superpowers," which we'll learn more about in chapter 6.

Also, living long and well should not be confused with living a good life. By many accounts, Picasso was not a nice person. People with horrific, murderous pasts have also lived long and well, while kind, loving people have ended their lives with Alzheimer's.

Nevertheless, given a choice, most people would prefer to chart the course of their lives to end up like Picasso, living independently, staying sharp, engaging with others, finding new avenues of meaningful and purposeful activity, and experiencing a quick death. We'll learn a few secrets of success that researchers have discovered from people who live long and well—called Super-Agers—in chapter 7.

Now we have an idea of what brain training success looks like: it means getting better with age and *living long and well*, like Picasso. To achieve this outcome, we need to do what we can to maintain neuroplasticity by managing our brain assets wisely throughout life's ups and downs.

However, our brain is not an object. We can't control it in the same way we would manage financial assets, like dollar bills, gold coin, or real estate. It is a living organ, built of flesh and blood, with a job to do. To protect neuroplasticity, we must stay out of our brain's way. So we'll continue with our voyage of discovery by learning a little about our brain's back story and warranty conditions.

A happy life is one spent learning, earning, and yearning.
LILLIAN GISH

Engagement questions

1. Have you ever been confused by media reports about brain health or Alzheimer's? If so, what do you find confusing?

2. What factors do you think have contributed the most to the rise in neurological disorders at all ages in the United States over the past thirty years? If you live outside of the United States, what neurological conditions are most common where you live?

3. Have you ever wondered if you were "losing it?" If so, what were the symptoms that concerned you?

4. Is there a pursuit that you hope to begin or return to in the future? If so, what attracts you to this activity?

5. Who do you know who has lived long and well until a ripe old age? What attitudes and habits do you think helped them do that?

6. Have you known anyone with Alzheimer's disease? How was their lifestyle similar to or different from that of someone you know who lived long and well?

7. Do you hope to live long and well? If so, what lifestyle choices and habits do you think are helping and hindering you in pursuing this outcome?

CHAPTER 2 A Brain for All Ages

 Look deep, deep into nature, and then you will understand everything better. ALBERT EINSTEIN

Your brain knows a heck of a lot about you, but how much do you know about your brain? Most people I meet know more about their car than they know about their brain. For example, many people still believe these outdated myths about our brain:

* We only use 10 percent of our brain.
* A normal brain declines with age.
* Advanced cognitive functions such as reasoning do not involve emotions.
* Thoughts and feelings do not alter brain chemistry.
* The rate of Alzheimer's disease is on the rise in the United States.

Perhaps because of this neuro-ignorance, many people are quick to sell our brain short. People over forty often think their brain is declining with age. It *embarrasses* them when it doesn't remember things fast enough. Sometimes people even diss their brains with remarks like "Oh, my stupid brain" or "My brain isn't working very well."

Worst of all, our brain has become the victim of identity theft. The dictionary states that a brainy person is someone with a well-developed intellect, as if the brain's reason for being is to produce the type of analytical ability measured by an intelligence quotient (IQ) test. However, our history as a species suggests that another kind of "intelligence" accounts for our brain's triumph over extinction (so far).

To profit from brain training, we will now get to know our brain a little better, and show a little respect for what it has done—and what it can do—for the human species and for each one of us.

21

our inner Grand canyon

If we were studying to become brain surgeons, we would get to know the brain by studying it from different scientific perspectives: genetic, molecular, structural, chemical, biological, functional, and so on. However, this approach is too complex for our purposes, so I have made up one just for us. We will learn more about our brain by considering its life story.

Here in Arizona, we have one of the greatest storytellers in the world: the Grand Canyon. Every year, some 5 million people from all over the world visit Arizona to learn more about the Grand Canyon's story.

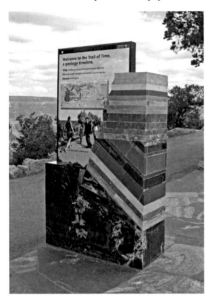

At the canyon's South Rim, a series of stations along a walking trail, called the Trail of Time, reveals two billion years of geological history. This exhibit allows people of all ages to stroll along, enjoying the magnificent view while discovering how and when the Grand Canyon's layers formed and how the rocks from these layers look and feel.

Unfortunately, we can't see or feel our brain's layers, so we'll have to improvise by taking a mental excursion along a Trail of Time

Figure 2.1. Entrance to the Trail of Time exhibit at the South Rim of the Grand Canyon.

to discover the past of our inner Grand Canyon, our brain.

Some four billion years ago, Mother Nature began birthing the first life on earth, invisible single-celled organisms. No one really knows how she pulled off this amazing feat. However, she endowed these little critters with abilities to counteract *entropy* (disorder) to stay alive, including:

Autonomy: the ability to manage and replicate oneself.

Movement: the ability to change physical location.

Spontaneity: the ability to respond to inner impulses.

Living organisms passed on these crucial survival abilities through their genes. Over time, many additional helpful tips and techniques for working around entropy were embedded in RNA and DNA and bequeathed through genes as well.

Our brain's fantastic voyage began some seven hundred million years ago. A simple multicellular critter like a jellyfish developed cells that could communicate with each other about the external environment by exchanging chemical signals called *neurotransmitters.* Some of the earliest neurotransmitters are still with us today, including *glutamate* (excitation), *GABA* (inhibition), *acetylcholine* (alertness), *dopamine* (pain or pleasure), *serotonin* (social activity), and *melatonin* (*circadian rhythms*).

These talkative cells were the earliest neurons, a term derived from the Greek word for "nerve" or "sinew." By figuring out what was up and sharing that information with the rest of the body through a network of physical channels called *nerves*, neurons could turn environmental cues into "news I can use" to guide an organism's behavior.

This inside information was so valuable to survival that neurons got a promotion and an office with a view. Some five hundred million years ago, a team of neurons formed the first brain in a fish. Protected by a skull and attached to a backbone, this spongy, self-managing organ operated as the chief executive officer for the body, exchanging messages with every cell via a *central nervous system.*

Appointing the brain as CEO of the body was a risky evolutionary gamble because it is a very high-maintenance organ. A brain that consumed more resources than it was worth would jeopardize the survival of an animal and its species. So brains had to justify their existence by improving the animal's ability to stay alive and reproduce. Fortunately, brains figured out how to add value by enhancing animals' performance of the four Fs: feeding, fighting, fleeing, and fornicating.

As a result, brains have been getting bigger and better ever since. To improve communication inside the body, neurons (or cells similar to them) also developed eventually in the eyes, spinal nerves, muscles, heart, adrenal glands, and gut—and maybe other places we don't even know about yet.

In building brains, Mother Nature has been equally passionate about employing the opposing forces of experimentation and efficiency. Millions of years of evolutionary trial and error have honed a wide variety of brain structures. Once a structure arose that did the job, it was shared by many species and became "highly conserved," becoming more and more effective and powerful as time went by.

As a result of Mother Nature's fondness for genetic recycling, every structure in the human brain can be found in the brains of other animals. Another characteristic our brain shares with other animals is bilateral specialization. Every structure in the brain appears in duplicate form: one in the left hemisphere to govern the right side of the body, and another in the right side to govern the left side of the body. The only structure that is not duplicated is the pineal gland, located in the middle of the brain. This melatonin-producing structure was part of the earliest brains, charged with managing the sleep-wake cycle and many other important activities.

Figure 2.2 indicates some of the major structures that are found in our brain and a rough estimate of when they became ready for prime time—revealing our own inner Grand Canyon. This is the inside story of how our brain came to be as we find it today.

In the 1960s, the neuroscientist Paul Maclean attempted to explain the similarities between human and animal brains with a theory called the triune brain. This theory identified three areas of the human brain: the reptilian complex (brain stem and cerebellum); the paleomammalian complex (limbic system); and the neomammalian complex (neocortex). The theory viewed these structures as sequentially developed and working in opposition at times, particularly with regard to morality.

Since Maclean's work, subsequent technological innovations, including fMRI (functional magnetic resonance imaging), have proved that the human brain is far more integrated than was thought in the 1960s. The reptilian, mammalian, and neomammalian structures in our brain are so closely coordinated that it is difficult to think of them as separate or opposing areas.

For example, the "switch" that flicks consciousness on or off involves coordinated activity by the brain stem, thalamus, hypothalamus, and

500 MILLION YEARS AGO:
Fish
Structures for cold-blooded living in the sea

- Basal ganglia
- Brain stem
- Cerebellum
- Cerebrum
- Cranial nerves (10)
- Olfactory bulb
- Pineal gland
- Spinal cord

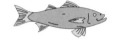

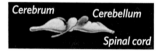

380 MILLION YEARS AGO:
Reptiles
Adaptations to living on land

- Cranial nerves (12)
- Expanded sensory and motor abilities

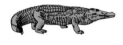

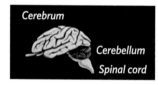

300 MILLION YEARS AGO:
Mammals
Structures for emotions and social living

- Limbic system
- Neocortex

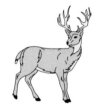

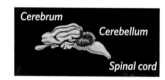

20 MILLION YEARS AGO:
Primates, cetaceans, elephants
Structure for advanced social communication

- Spindle (von Economo) neurons

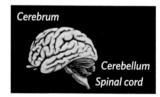

200,000 YEARS AGO:
Humans
Circuit for autobiographical sense of self

- Default network

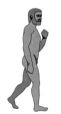

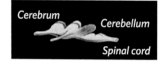

Figure 2.2. Our inner Grand Canyon: a snapshot of how the human brain has evolved.

anterior cingulate cortex. These primitive areas of our brain control access to our most advanced capacity, self-consciousness.

In addition, decades of research have confirmed limits to the similarities of brains. A particular structure and the neurotransmitters that engage it do not necessarily have the same function from species to species. This means that brain research findings are not always transferable from model animals to humans.

our Brain the Hero

If I could share a cup of coffee with Mother Nature, I would love to ask her why she worked so hard for so long to make our brain as it is today. I would also ask about some unthinkably cruel moves that have gotten us to where we are today. For instance, what was Mother Nature thinking when the earliest mammals—nursing, whimpering, furry, cute, cuddly, affectionate, playful, fearful, loyal, vulnerable, tiny little animals similar to a shrew—were placed at the feet of the monstrous dinosaurs over 200 million years ago?

Evolutionary process may be heartless at times, but it has been very, very good to us. Some two hundred thousand years ago, our species, *Homo sapiens sapiens,* showed up in the life-on-earth scene, equipped with a first-class brain carrying some very impressive features. The cornerstone of the human brain's phenomenal powers is the orchestration of an autobiographical self that persists seamlessly over a lifetime and gets better with age.

But the downside of our high-powered brain is that it guzzles resources like a car that gets one mile to the gallon. Although it weighs only three pounds, our brain hogs 20 to 30 percent of the calories, oxygen, and water our body takes in. In times of plenty, such extravagant consumption could be overlooked. But could the human brain really justify these resources in hard times?

About seventy thousand years ago, the forces of nature administered the greatest test to date of our brain's ability to pull its own weight. Although it's not clear exactly what happened, a deadly disaster occurred, possibly a massive volcanic eruption of Mount Koba in Indonesia. The

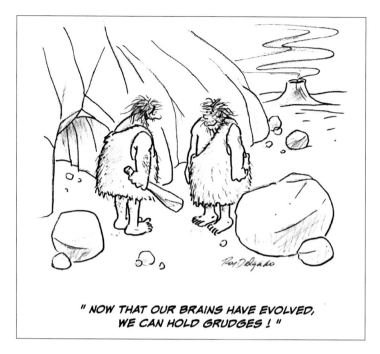

" NOW THAT OUR BRAINS HAVE EVOLVED,
WE CAN HOLD GRUDGES ! "

lava really hit the fan, quickly triggering a volcanic winter that lasted for years.

In the aftermath of this environmental catastrophe, temperatures dropped suddenly and food became scarce, even in the tropics. The human population died off, dropping to a few thousand breeding pairs living in groups close to each other in sub-Saharan Africa.

Human genome research has revealed that this close call created an unusual pattern in our DNA, referred to as a genetic bottleneck. All humans alive today have descended from this small clan of savvy survivors. Each of us is 99.9 percent biochemically similar to any other human, regardless of apparent differences. This level of genetic similarity is unknown in other species.

This narrow victory was our brain's finest hour! We would not be here if our brain had not pulled its weight and bailed us out. Somehow our ancestors partnered with our brain to cheat extinction without the aid of books, computers, college, smartphones, artificial intelligence, or anything else we associate with "intelligence" today.

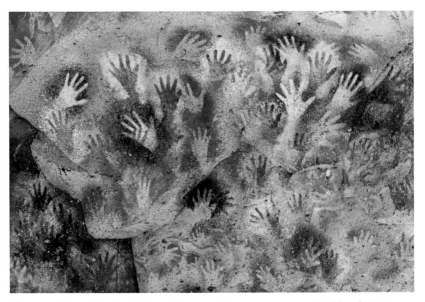

Figure 2.3. Cave of the Hands, Argentina, created 10,000 years ago. Most handprints in ancient cave drawings were made by women.

So in this time of hardship, what kept humans from destroying each other in a downward spiral of fear and violence that would have kept their nervous systems in permanent overdrive? What was the magic trick our brain used to survive the worst times we have ever faced, and then subsequently climb to new cultural heights?

We know the answer wasn't food, as that was in short supply. And we know that it wasn't exercise, as these survivors were already getting plenty of exercise looking for food. Even today, findings confirm that optimal levels of nutrition and exercise by themselves do not guarantee health or longevity.

Perhaps our ancestors stumbled upon some stress-busting activities that allowed them to blow off steam and trust each other. They had access to the same relaxation techniques that work for us today, including sex, breastfeeding, call and response, caring, chanting, cuddling, dancing, empathy, eye contact, forgiveness, friendship, generosity, hugging, intimacy, laughter, love, magical thinking, music, nurturing, praying, reciprocity, ritual, romance, sex, sharing, singing, smiling, talking, teamwork, touching, and, of course, sex.

Faced with extinction some seventy thousand years ago, perhaps our brain figured out how to maximize the biochemical upside of all of our prosocial neurotransmitters, including **oxytocin, vasopressin,** and serotonin. This magic trick allowed our ancestors to master toxic emotions and use **rationality** to preserve the community with wisdom and justice.

Once our ancestors figured out how to *control their thoughts* to keep toxic stress and violence in line, they were able to find ways to use our species' innate ability for technology to find new food sources and preserve the species. But to do this, rationality and technology had to serve the common good, not destroy it.

Whatever happened 70,000 years ago, it was a huge success. Ever since this pivotal time, we have managed to come up with one killer application after another for our brain:

Migration out of Africa:	60,000 years ago
Music:	43,000 years ago
Art:	40,000 years ago
Domestication of wolves:	25,000 years ago
Agriculture:	15,000 years ago
Spiritual ritual:	11,000 years ago
Modern languages:	10,000 years ago
Calendar:	7,000 years ago
Mathematics:	5,400 years ago
Writing:	5,000 years ago
Meditation:	3,000 years ago
Drama:	2,700 years ago
Science:	2,600 years ago
Birth control pill:	50 years ago

This ancient success over extinction passed on to us a brain that is even more hungry for love and service to others than for food. For better or worse, our social interactions sculpt our brain tissue, gut bacteria, and telomeres from the womb to the grave—even more than food, exercise, or technology does.

The essence of this unique social interdependence is characterized by Archbishop Desmond Tutu as the African concept of *Ubuntu:* "One

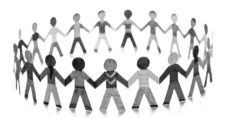

of the sayings in our country is Ubuntu—the essence of being human. Ubuntu speaks particularly about the fact that you can't exist as a human being in isolation. It speaks about our interconnectedness. You can't be human all by yourself, and when you have this quality—Ubuntu—you are known for your generosity."

As a result of our genetic back story, our brain is touchy about being without love and people for long periods. You never know when the next volcanic eruption might make the lava hit the fan again.

With this background in mind, let's explore how our brain develops over time to nurture social relationships and craft a unique human life.

A Brain for All stages

Today, we all carry the latest, greatest, new and improved version of the human brain (no extra charge for this valuable upgrade). Thanks to neuroplasticity, our brain develops throughout life in a way that reflects the lessons learned in keeping our species going through thick and thin for some two hundred thousand years.

Researchers have made great progress in understanding the brain's early stages of physiological development to support the treatment of childhood neurological diseases and disorders. However, healthy brain function, particularly in adulthood, has been studied less thoroughly. We will revisit this topic in chapter 7 for some exciting new research findings about people who age, like Picasso, to live long and well.

But our brain is only part of the story of whole-person maturity in a social context. As neuroscience has progressed in understanding our brain's physiological stages of development, social scientists have generated theories about psychological and spiritual development over the human life span. We will look more closely at this topic in chapter 6.

Figure 2.4 indicates the major objective of structural brain development: to bring on line brain circuits that enable sensory-motor skills, cognitive control, and default mode activity. Human **attachment** is the foundation for all of these circuits.

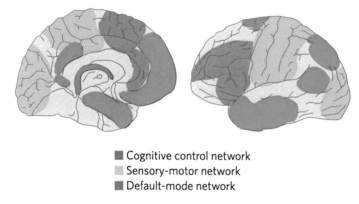

■ Cognitive control network
▢ Sensory-motor network
■ Default-mode network

Figure 2.4. Brain development aims to integrate the activities of three major networks: sensory-motor; cognitive control; and default mode.

However, brain development is a highly complicated subject that we are not going to cover in any detail here. We'll consider just the gist of how the human brain matures throughout life.

Overall, our brain's typical pattern of development follows a few general rules:

* *Bottom to top:* Foundational structures such as the brain stem, cerebellum, and basal ganglia develop first, and the lowest layers of the **cerebral cortex** develop before the upper layers. The sixth layer of the cerebral cortex, the outer layer that facilitates brain integration, is fully developed by around age 30.

* *Back to front:* Brain asset development roughly follows the order of where the structures are located, with the occipital and parietal lobes at the back finishing development first, followed by the temporal and frontal lobes.

* *Right to left:* The right hemisphere, associated with emotions and body awareness, is dominant for the first five years of life to enable attachment. The left hemisphere, associated with language and rationality, gradually comes up to speed between the ages of 6 and 12. An early sign of this transition and the brain's readiness to learn to read and write is a child's ability to recognize words that rhyme.

* *Outside to inside:* The outer (lateral) brain surfaces develop first, processing information and solving problems related to the outer world. The inner (medial) brain surfaces, charged mainly with processing the inner mental world of a person, develop most actively over age 40.

* *First in, last out:* The first brain assets to develop (occipital and parietal) are the last ones to be affected by dementia. The last brain assets to develop (temporal and frontal lobes) are the first to be affected by cognitive decline and dementia.

Now let's take a peek at what the brain does to support the major stages of our lives in a social context. The stages of life below correlate roughly with key stages of brain development, as well as the typical social roles played at each stage, based on the traditional extended-family lifestyle. The common markers for the end of each stage are indicated as well.

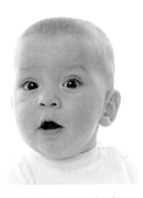

Stage 1: Heart, birth to age 12

Brain's priority: development of neurological foundation for emotional activity and sensory-motor skills to enable attachment, empathy, and trust

Traditional social role: childhood

A baby is born with close to a full complement of 100 billion neurons, which will be with the baby throughout life unless they die off, as neurons do not divide and reproduce themselves. The newborn's brain is a human attachment machine and has no interest in becoming a Baby Einstein. It correctly perceives behaviors such as grasping, smiling, and eye contact to be of more survival value than intelligence during early childhood.

Most brain development occurs after birth, mainly through the growth and pruning of synaptic connections between neurons, but also through the growth of new neurons (*neurogenesis*). By age 2, a child has some 500 trillion synaptic connections, about as many as the average adult.

However, most of the two-year-old's synaptic connections are not myelinated, making communication between neurons highly inefficient. *Myelin* is a fatty coating (sheath) on the neuron's *axon*, which acts like insulation to expedite the transmission of messages between neurons. On myelinated axons, messages travel at nearly three hundred miles per hour, but on unmyelinated axons they travel much more slowly. The myelination process continues through late adolescence.

Early brain development focuses on sensory processing, emotional responses, and motor skills to support basic attachment behaviors such as eye contact, laughing, listening, recognizing faces and voices, assessing emotions and intentions, smiling, talking, touching, and walking. By the age of eighteen months, an infant can use empathy to read emotional expressions; by age 2, a baby can use this information to decide whether to trust someone.

By ages 3–5, the neurological ground work for *theory of mind* skills (understanding mental states, associated with the default network) and cognitive control skills (executive functions) is in place. During this period, important activities that build a child's cognitive readiness for language include:

1. Call-and-response communication
2. Conversation
3. Imitation
4. Manipulating objects
5. Pattern recognition
6. Rituals
7. Understanding of shared symbols

Between ages 6 and 12, the brain is mobilized to learn language and generate a social *identity* (how the individual fits into the social context).

Sexual maturity occurs long before the brain is fully developed. While puberty often occurs between ages 11 and 14, the frontal lobe is not fully developed until ages 25–30—the age of grandparenthood in a tribal society.

Stage 1 typically culminates in puberty and coming-of-age social rituals.

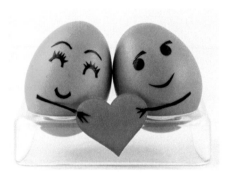

Stage 2: Mind, ages 12–40

Brain's priority: development of executive functions to perform roles in society

Traditional social roles: marriage, parenthood, and grandparenthood

In this stage, the brain works very hard to expand the frontal lobe's powers, known as *executive functions* (EF), a set of abilities that direct non-routinized behavior for self-determined goals. EF gives us the brain reins to steer our own behavior toward desirable outcomes that benefit our social group. We'll learn more about EF in chapter 6.

While EF connects our outer and inner worlds, the development process is uneven. Dominated by visual input and the lateral areas of the frontal lobe, the capacity for outer-oriented EF activity (cognitive control) matures first, in stage 2. This network of areas helps us to focus on extrinsic rewards, goals, judgment, objects, problem solving, and tasks as we find our place in society through family life, friendships, and work. The areas involved in inner-oriented EF mental activity (default mode) mature after age 40, in stage 3.

The outer-oriented and inner-oriented brain processing areas tend to be inversely correlated during this second stage of life, making it difficult for us to focus on tasks and emotions at the same time. Emotional activity can be challenging to understand and manage, easily leading to toxic emotions such as anger, frustration, and resentment that can trigger health and relationship problems.

In modern times, a work-life balance struggle is a common outcome toward the end of stage 2.

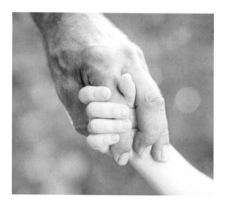

Stage 3: Spirit, age 40 through death

Brain's priority: integration of brain activity to generate wisdom

Traditional social roles: great-grandparenthood and tribal elder

As we approach stage 3, our default network and inner-oriented awareness and thinking become more active. The challenge is to be born again, from the inside out. Between ages 40 and 50, this transition in brain activity from an outer focus to an inner focus can be disruptive, perhaps connected to the midlife-crisis phenomenon.

The default network performs our brain's most advanced activity, and, not surprisingly, it uses the most energy. This inner-oriented network connects important hubs throughout the brain along the medial (inner) surfaces of the brain. The default network, in charge of our life story, gives us access to our most human qualities, especially theory of mind skills and wisdom.

After age 50, the cerebral cortex's memory center (the medial temporal lobe) becomes integrated with the default network. At this time, a noticeable increase occurs in nostalgia and thinking about one's past.

After this shift, the brain's focus is on integrating the activity of the inner- and outer-oriented networks, so that they become more positively correlated, working together rather than in opposition. The synchronized activity of these two networks creates more congruency between one's outer and inner worlds, yielding greater integrity and wisdom. The name of the human species, *Homo sapiens sapiens,* comes from the Latin words for "man" and "wisdom." Wisdom and its cohort, generativity, are the "gold" of the golden years.

At age 55, Elizabeth Taylor spoke about this stage 3 "trenaissance" during an interview with *Rolling Stone* magazine:

I've always been very aware of the inner me that has nothing to do with the physical me. . . . Eventually the inner you shapes the outer you, especially when you reach a certain age, and you have been given the same features as everybody else, God has arranged them in a certain way. But around 40 the inner you actually chisels your features. . . . Life is to be embraced and enveloped. Surgeons and knives have nothing to do with it. It has to do with a connection with nature, God, your inner being—whatever you want to call it—it's being in contact with yourself and allowing yourself, allowing God, to mold you.

Stage 3 culminates at death, completing our brain's active duty to both the individual and our species.

A Hollywood Ending

As a result of this three-stage pattern of development, our brain has different strengths at different ages. A five-year-old brain is highly creative and quick to learn from others; a thirty-year-old brain is near the height of its powers with regard to processing speed and reaction time; and the over-fifty brain has vast memory stores to share wisdom and solve problems for the common good. Thus, our brain's performance cannot be properly benchmarked using the same criteria for all ages.

However, these stages are a guideline only. If your life doesn't unfold in the order above, don't worry about it. The culture (family, town, workplace, and country) you live in has a huge impact on brain development at different stages.

Besides, when our brain is so multitalented and highly adaptive, there is no reason to take a "one size fits all" approach to the human journey for all 7 billion people on earth. Neuroplasticity continues throughout life in a healthy brain, allowing for tremendous flexibility and adaptability. An attachment disorder in childhood can be straightened out through healthy relationships later in life. Some people focus on spiritual development in stage 2, and some focus on parenting in stage 3.

What's most important is to keep an eye on the end game. The integration of our experiences into an autobiographical self is the ultimate human experience that our brain can deliver, regardless of how we get there. Balance between our inner and outer worlds allows us to be in the world, but not of the world, blessed with a brain and a life that get better with age and an unquenchable *joie de vivre* (joy of living).

The personal reward for achieving this balance between the outer and inner worlds is the triumphant sense of a life well lived, like a Hollywood ending to an autobiography. As the Romans said, *Per aspera ad astra,* or "Through difficulties to the stars."

Now that we are better acquainted with our brain, we can continue on our way to discover a hidden treasure: our brain assets.

The future belongs to those who believe
in the beauty of their dreams.
ELEANOR ROOSEVELT

Engagement questions

1. Did you think that any of the brain myths at the beginning of this chapter were true? Which ones and why?

2. What surprises you most about our brain's back story?

3. What do you think happened seventy thousand years ago that allowed the human species to escape extinction?

4. What stage of life are you in now? Is there any unfinished business in your life from earlier stages?

5. How does your social life help or hinder your health at this point in your life?

6. What major challenges have you faced in balancing your outer and inner worlds? Who has provided a good model for you on how to do this?

7. Who has served as an important source of wisdom for you?

8. If you are in stage 3 (over 40 years old), how have you shared your wisdom with the next generation? What opportunities for sharing your wisdom do you hope to pursue in the future?

CHAPTER 3

Brain Assets

 The meeting of two personalities is like the contact of two chemical substances; if there is any reaction, both are transformed. CARL JUNG

During my early days as a brain coach, I took a methodical approach to explaining the brain and how it works. I knew that some words I had learned, such as *telencephalon, diencephalon,* and *mesencephalon,* were not going to work for my audience. I figured words like *brain stem, cerebellum, limbic system, occipital lobe,* and *oxytocin* would work.

Boy, was I wrong. My audience, people over fifty who wanted to improve brain fitness, generally had little background in science. They found it difficult to learn the jargon of neuroscience, let alone apply it in daily life. They also struggled with discussing emotions or unconscious mental activity.

Then one day a woman raised her hand in class and said, "This is so complicated, is there any way we can just take a pill to make this all work right?" That was when I knew something had to change in my teaching approach.

No one can successfully act on information without a clear image of the desired outcome embedded in the brain. I had learned this same lesson in financial services sales: confusion breeds inaction, and confusion comes easily to even the smartest people when encountering new information.

Since my audience was well-heeled, it occurred to me that the analogy of money might make the scientific information easier to take in—and even get excited about. When it comes to our brain, the exciting news is that *everyone* is a billionaire many times over!

My audience did not need a scientific background or even a college degree to think of the brain as a portfolio of assets that needed to be rebalanced from time to time to get big returns. Over time, I developed this approach to simplify the most complex structure in the universe for daily management and use.

Defining Brain Assets

Now let's examine our portfolio of brain assets. Photographs and images of the brain commonly depict a pinkish, wrinkled structure: the *cerebral cortex*, the outermost layer of our brain that is only 3–4 millimeters thick (less than 1/6 of an inch). The five brain assets we will become acquainted with are located in the cerebral cortex, associated with our most advanced cognitive abilities.

As we learned in chapter 2, the cerebral cortex evolved after the lower, more primitive brain structures below. However, this upper region of our brain is dependent on the lower structures to do its job, just as the walls and roof of a building cannot stand without the invisible foundation that lies underground.

For the sake of simplicity, we are going to focus on learning more about the outer wrinkly area, the cerebral cortex. However, since the lower areas are the gateway to consciousness and are implicated in many neurological disorders, we will at least introduce these areas so you are acquainted with them.

Figure 3.1 indicates several efficient and powerful structures in our brain that underwrite our most basic activities. Located at the bottom center of the brain, the **brain stem** is largely involved in maintaining vital functions and homeostasis. The **cerebellum**, Latin for "little brain," is a relatively large, mysterious structure at the back of the brain dedicated to refining voluntary movement and possibly other important functions such as memory.

Situated at the center of the brain, the **thalamus** is similar to an air traffic control tower for incoming sensory information. It directs the information to the appropriate brain areas for further processing, with the exception of smells, which go directly to the olfactory cortex.

Centrally located at the base of the front of the brain, the **basal ganglia** are a collection of structures that underwrite brain activity related to emotion, cognition, voluntary movement, procedural learning, and

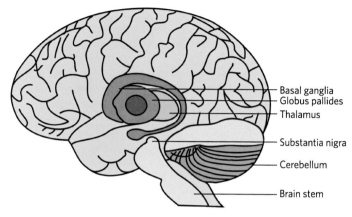

Basal ganglia
Globus pallides
Thalamus

Substantia nigra

Cerebellum

Brain stem

Figure 3.1. Basal ganglia and nearby structures form the neurological foundation of higher cognitive functions.

certain habits such as teeth-grinding during sleep. The substantia nigra, near the top of the brain stem, produces most of the brain's dopamine, required for all voluntary movement. This is the main area affected by Parkinson's disease.

Figure 3.2 maps out the *limbic system*, the mammalian brain innovation which we met in chapter 2. Important structures related to emotions (amygdala and insula), homeostasis (hypothalamus and pituitary gland), and memory (*hippocampus*) are included in the limbic system.

As we learned earlier, the hypothalamus and pituitary initiate the stress-response system, and the hippocampus is impaired in the early stages of Alzheimer's disease. We will learn more about another important limbic structure called the cingulate cortex in chapter 6.

Now we'll get to know our brain assets. The first four brain assets we review are the different territories, or lobes, of the cerebral cortex: parietal, occipital, temporal, and frontal. These large regions, identified over one hundred years ago, are named for the adjacent bones of the skull that contain them.

In figure 3.3, the territory included in each of these four brain assets is indicated by color: frontal (blue), occipital (green), parietal (yellow), and temporal (pink). The numbered regions refer to the Brodmann's areas included in each brain asset. The German neurologist Korbinian Brodmann (1868–1918) mapped the cerebral cortex into structurally distinct

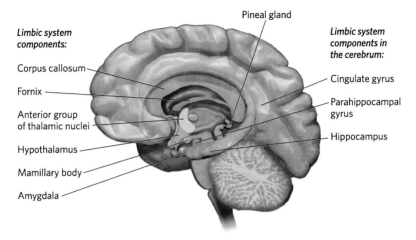

Pineal gland

Limbic system
components:

Corpus callosum

Fornix

Anterior group
of thalamic nuclei

Hypothalamus

Mamillary body

Amygdala

Limbic system
components in
the cerebrum:

Cingulate gyrus

Parahippocampal
gyrus

Hippocampus

Figure 3.2. The limbic system integrates lower brain structures with the upper cerebral cortex.

regions that have proved to be useful in identifying the functions of particular brain areas. Each region has a number assigned.

The fifth brain asset I present here, the default network, is not a specific structure but the coordinated activity of several key brain structures, including major hubs in the parietal, temporal, and frontal lobes (more on this later in the chapter). The occipital lobe, occupied mainly with visual activity and the outer world, is *not* part of the default network, which is primarily involved with the inner mental world of an individual and memory retrieval.

The default network is one of dozens of neural networks, or teams of neurons, that perform specific roles in the brain. I emphasize the default network because it is the network most affected by Alzheimer's disease and thus merits special attention from anyone interested in growing their brain wealth to get better with age.

As indicated in figure 3.3, each of our five brain assets covers territory on both sides of our brain, the left and right hemispheres. As we learned in chapter 2, all structures in our brain except for the pineal gland (shown in figure 3.2) are duplicated in each hemisphere.

The two hemispheres have specialized, complementary functions. Most importantly, the left brain controls the right side of the body, and the right brain controls the left side of the body. Therefore, all motor

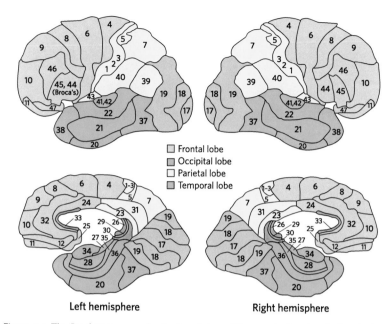

Figure 3.3. The Brodmann areas for the four lobes of the cerebral cortex, by hemisphere.

output (movement) requires both sides of our brain to work together. Our brain functions best when the two sides work together, and motor output is crucial to the teamwork between hemispheres.

Because of their specialized functions, the two hemispheres are also associated with different types of mental activity, as reflected in the comparison of several qualities in figure 3.4.

As this list indicates, both sides have valuable functions, and we operate at our best when we have access to both sides. I think of our left and right hemispheres working together like the keys of the piano. A song played with all white keys sounds hollow and lacks depth, like the left hemisphere working without the right. A song played with all black keys sounds brooding and sad, like a right hemisphere working without the left. Together, the left and right sides of our brain complement each other to make an endless variety of beautiful harmonies.

тhe whole-person вrain

While some people may be more adept at using one side of the brain than the other, the goal is to have access to all these abilities when needed. In

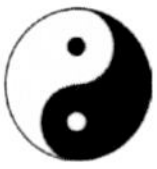

Left Hemisphere		Right Hemisphere
Abstract information		Concrete information
Analysis		Synthesis
Approach		Retreat
Clarity		Mystery
Complexity		Simplicity
Details		Patterns
Duty		Passion
Emotional regulation		Emotional expression
Judging		Perceiving
Linear thought		Lateral thought
Objective thought		Subjective thought
Preparation		Spontaneity
Probabilities		Possibilities
Processing new information		Habit formation
Rationality		Intuition
Remembering names		Remembering faces
Self-interest		Relatedness
Sexual desire		Romance
Speaking		Listening
Time—*chronos* (what time is it?)		Time—*kairos* (what is it time for?)
Using objects		Connecting with people
Work		Play
Verbal language		Body language
Yang		Yin

Figure 3.4. The specialized functions of the left and right hemispheres are complementary.

order to ensure this outcome, the two sides of our brain share information. The main pathway of communication between the two hemispheres is a thick band of synaptic connections called the *corpus callosum* (Latin for "hard body"), located between the two hemispheres near the center of the brain (see figure 3.2).

However, the split-brain research of the 1960s and 1970s, for which Roger Sperry earned a Nobel Prize in 1981, proved that communication between the two hemispheres takes place in various areas of our brain and is not limited to the corpus callosum.

I also learned this firsthand from meeting two unusual young men, each of whom had undergone a hemispherectomy. The first young man, Albert, in his early twenties, had had the entire left side of his cerebral cortex removed by neurosurgeons. Albert had suffered from severe seizures and would have needed some seventy different medications every day to try and control them. The surgery was a desperate attempt to find a better way to control the seizures.

Despite this radical surgery, Albert led a pretty normal life, holding down a job, sharing an apartment with friends, and playing the guitar. And he had a great sense of humor! At the neuroscience conference where he was a guest speaker, Albert acknowledged some challenges, such as difficulty with managing emotions and a limited vocabulary (tasks typically performed by the left brain). He described a technique he used to manage anger: thinking of good memories as wrapped presents on a shelf at the back of his mind that he could retrieve and unwrap when he felt angry.

Some years later, I met a seventeen-year-old high school student named Robert. Like Albert, Robert had had a hemispherectomy to control seizures, but in his case surgeons had removed the right side of his cortex. Robert seemed to have some of the social difficulties associated with autism spectrum disorder—as one might expect, since the right brain is specialized for emotional processing, facial recognition, and interpersonal interaction.

But once we got talking about Robert's favorite subject—music—he warmed right up, looked me in the eyes, and smiled frequently. He had an encyclopedic knowledge of the songs by his favorite artists, and he volunteered as a disc jockey in addition to attending high school.

My direct experiences with Albert and Robert convinced me that our brain's capacity for teamwork and neuroplasticity can overcome just about any challenge we might face. And if Albert and Robert can function so well with only half a brain, the rest of us are leaving a whole lot of money on the table in terms of brain performance. We should all be working to access our whole brain—left, right, back, front, bottom, top—to act as a whole person and get where we want to go in life.

The stories of Albert and Robert suggest that the blueprint for constructing a whole-person member of the human species is present in our whole being, not limited to certain brain structures or body parts. Perhaps this blueprint is contained in our RNA and DNA. If so, our whole-person identity is present in every cell of the body, including but not limited to our brain.

A whole-person, real-life understanding of our brain has been elusive. Scientists in the areas of neuroscience, *cognitive neuroscience*, psychology, and psychiatry don't often see things the same way, let alone integrate their research findings.

In particular, distinguishing between the mind and the brain continues to be a challenge for many researchers. At a conference last year, a leading cognitive neuroscience researcher shared that he and a group of colleagues got together one day to come up with a working definition of *mind*. After three hours, they still didn't have one. They probably would not have found it any easier to arrive at a working definition of *spirit*.

For our purposes here, we will look at the brain from a whole-person perspective, an approach rooted in cognitive neuroscience but not limited to it. To keep things simple, we will think of the brain as a body part that mediates our experience of life: body, mind, spirit, heart, and soul.

Body, the source of feelings, is a physical entity that exists both in time and in the three dimensions of space (height, length, and width).

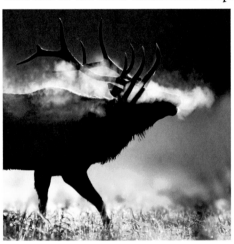 I use **mind** to refer primarily to thinking, the mind's most important capability. *Spirit,* from the Latin word for breath, refers to an awareness of the life force within and around us. Heart is the seat of feelings and will, and **soul** is the unique, whole-person blueprint that is built out through our life story.

We will explore our brain assets by considering their qualities and the ways they influence our whole-person experience of life. Even though we are analyzing our brain's different physical parts, it's important to remember that it remains a single, integrated entity. Brain assets are like the facets of a jewel that can be viewed individually, but not separated from the jewel.

Remember, all of us have all five of these brain assets. And even if a brain area is damaged or missing, our brain retains some ability to perform the duties of these assets: like a financial portfolio, our brain assets can be redistributed and rebalanced. The key is to employ our full mental range of motion and appreciate the beauty of our existence in manifold ways.

Below is a brief introduction to our brain assets as I understand them, and how they have been expressed in our experience of life as individuals and in culture. In chapter 4, we will look more closely at what they can do for us and how to manage them as a portfolio of assets invested for long-term growth.

As long as our brain is a mystery, the universe,
the reflection of the structure of the brain,
will also be a mystery.
SANTIAGO RAMÓN Y CAJAL

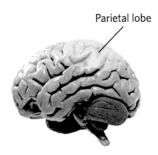

Parietal lobe

Brain Asset 1: Parietal Lobe

Qualities

Subsections: **Somatosensory cortex, superior parietal lobule, inferior parietal lobule, precuneus**

Engaged by: **Aggression, novelty, physical sensations, risk, sexuality, spontaneity, technology, tools**

Expert at processing: **Touch (sensing kinetic energy)**

Focus: **The unknown**

Mental range of motion: **Adventure**

Preferred outcomes: **Excitement, fun, solving concrete problems, tangible rewards, thrills**

Role in culture: **Migration**

Values: **Courage, freedom, heroism, independence, pragmatism**

Vulnerability: **Freedom without responsibility**

Quips

Bring it on.

"Can't" is a coward too lazy to try.

Don't tread on me.

Give me liberty or give me death.

If you can't handle the heat, get out of the kitchen.

If you find a fork in the road, take it.

I did it my way.

I've seen a lot of trouble that never was.

If you can be lost, you can also be found.

Nothing ventured, nothing gained.

No pain, no gain.

When the going gets tough, the tough get going.

Analogues

Biological process: Innovation

Chemical element: Nitrogen

Force of nature: Strong nuclear force

Figures in Greek mythology: Ares, Artemis, Hephaistos, Hermes

Keirsey temperament: Artisan

Military: Tactics

Wizard of Oz character: Cowardly Lion

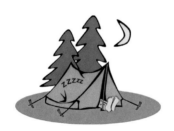

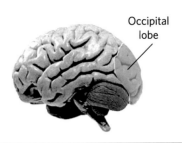

Occipital lobe

Brain Asset 2: occipital Lobe

Qualities

Subsections: Primary visual cortex, secondary visual cortex, cuneus

Engaged by: Beauty, competition, desire, images, ritual, routine, rules, structure, tasks, threats

Expert at processing: Vision (sensing light energy)

Focus: The score

Mental range of motion: Achievement

Preferred outcomes: Cooperation, socially defined rewards, stability, status, teamwork, winning

Role in culture: Preserving tradition

Values: Closure, control, efficiency, loyalty, political pragmatism, social order, security

Vulnerability: Order without freedom

Quips

A picture is worth a thousand words.
A place for everything, everything in its place.
Better the devil you know than the one you don't.
Don't reinvent the wheel.
Don't upset the apple cart.
Get your ducks in a row.
Good fences make good neighbors.
Living well is the best revenge.
No surprises.
Not on my watch.
Politics makes strange bedfellows.
Seeing is believing.
The ends justify the means.
Winning isn't everything; it's the only thing.

Analogues

Biological process: Replication
Chemical element: Oxygen
Force of nature: Electromagnetism
Figures in Greek mythology: Aphrodite, Hera, Poseidon
Keirsey temperament: Guardian
Military: Operations
Wizard of Oz character: Wizard

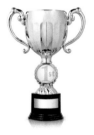

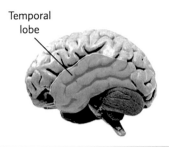

Temporal
lobe

Brain Asset 3: Temporal Lobe

Qualities

Subsections: Auditory cortex, fusiform, gustatory cortex, limbic system, olfactory cortex, temporal pole, *Wernicke's area*

Engaged by: Dreams, emotional expression, fantasy, identification of objects and people, personal interaction, memory storage, mentoring, music, spirituality, storytelling

Expert at processing: Hearing (sensing sound energy), smell (sensing airborne odorant molecules), taste (detecting water-based odorant molecules)

Focus: The heart

Mental range of motion: Attachment

Preferred outcomes: Affiliation, affirmation, collaboration, communication, friendship, helping others, praise, social recognition

Role in culture: Language

Values: Devotion, fulfillment, happiness, harmony, interdependence, passion, timing, truth

Vulnerability: Passion without rationality

Quips

All the world's a stage.
Follow your heart.
Home is where the heart is.
Music is the language of the soul.
The pen is mightier than the sword.
People matter more than things.
A rose by any other name would smell as sweet.
The truth will set you free.
Those who live by the sword, die by the sword.
Timing is everything.
You can't be human by yourself.
Why can't we all just get along?
United we stand, divided we fall.

Analogues

Biological process: Transformation
Chemical element: Carbon
Force of nature: Weak nuclear force
Figures in Greek mythology: Apollo, Demeter, Dionysus, Hestia
Keirsey temperament: Idealist
Military: Diplomacy
Wizard of Oz character: Tin Man

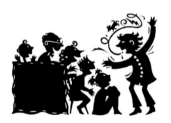

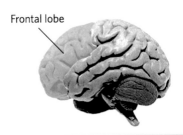

Frontal lobe

Brain Asset 4: Frontal Lobe

Qualities

Subsections: ***Broca's area***, frontal eye fields, motor cortex, orbitofrontal cortex, prefrontal cortex, premotor cortex, supplementary motor area

Engaged by: Big picture, conflicts, curiosity, decisions, envisioning the future, goals, imagination, learning, nonroutine behavior, planning, prediction, self-determination, vision, wonder

Expert at processing: Movement, speech, working memory

Focus: The future

Mental range of motion: Adaptation

Preferred outcomes: The common good, fairness, logic, self-mastery, understanding origins, victory

Role in culture: Justice

Values: Autonomy, clarity, confidence, faith, hope, inspiration, optimism, perspective, rationality

Vulnerability: Rationality without mercy

Quips

An ounce of prevention is worth a pound of cure.
Begin with the end in mind.
If you don't know where you're going, any road will take you there.
Just because we can doesn't mean we should.
Look before you leap.
The past is prologue.
The plan is nothing; the planning is everything.
Those who don't learn from history are doomed to repeat it.
You can't solve problems with the same thinking that created them.
You have to believe it to see it.
You can lose a battle but still win the war.
What goes around, comes around.

Analogues

Biological process: Execution
Chemical element: Hydrogen
Force of nature: Gravity
Figures in Greek mythology: Athena, Zeus
Keirsey temperament: Rationalist
Military: Strategy
Wizard of Oz character: Scarecrow

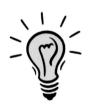

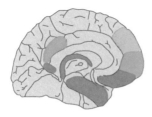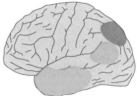

Brain Asset 5: Default Network

Qualities

Subregions: Hippocampus, medial prefrontal cortex, inferior parietal cortex, lateral temporal cortex, medial temporal lobe, posterior cingulate cortex/retrosplinal cortex, precuneus

Engaged by: Daydreaming, empathy, humor, identity, intimacy, intrinsic motivation, legacy, memory retrieval, morality, personal narrative, self-expression, understanding mental states, yearning

Expert at processing: Consciousness

Focus: Relationships

Mental range of motion: Autobiography

Preferred outcomes: Forgiveness, gratitude, heroism, honesty, inner peace, mutuality, purpose, righteousness, self-awareness, serving others

Role in culture: Wisdom

Values: Authenticity, biophilia, humility, integrity, love, mercy, patience, persistence, personal meaning, righteousness, self-respect

Vulnerability: Love without suffering

Quips

Be yourself; everyone else is already taken.
A friend in need is a friend indeed.
Get a life.
Know thyself.
Love makes the world go 'round.
Love your neighbor as yourself.
Money can't buy me love.
Speak truth to power.
To thine own self be true.
What good is it to gain the world and lose your own self?
The unexamined life is not worth living for a human being.
It is better to have loved and lost than never to have loved at all.

Analogues

Biological process: Integration
Chemical element: Phosphorus
Force of nature: Neutrinos
Figures in Greek mythology: Odysseus, Prometheus
Keirsey temperament: The individual
Military: The hero
Wizard of Oz character: Dorothy

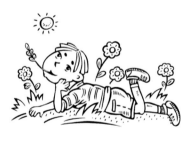

Engagement Questions

1. Do you prefer to use one cerebral hemisphere over the other? If so, which one and why?

2. Do you know someone who prefers to use the opposite hemisphere from you? How does this difference help or hinder your relationship?

3. Were you familiar with any of the brain assets before reading *Better with Age?* If so, which ones and why?

4. Which of the five brain assets do you work the hardest and the least? What models and experiences have encouraged you to do this?

5. Who do you know who has been especially strong in using one or two particular brain assets? What do you admire about them?

6. Do you think you are "leaving a whole lot of money on the table" in terms of brain performance"? Why or why not?

7. Is there another brain asset you wish we had? What would it do?

CHAPTER 4

The Brain Portfolio Tool

 There are three things extremely hard: steel, a diamond, and to know one's self. BENJAMIN FRANKLIN

In chapter 3, we became acquainted with our brain assets and their differing qualities. Now we'll learn a simple way to manage our own brain assets for long-term growth to get better with age, using the Brain Portfolio Tool.

First, let me share the story of how this tool came to be. The Brain Portfolio Tool arose from my own personal brain-training adventures. I began trying to train my brain in 2004, when I was forty-six years old, just after my book *The Richest of Fare* had been published. In chapter 4 of *The Richest of Fare*, I had written about the evolution of our brain and consciousness and briefly discussed the cerebral cortex. This effort sparked my interest in learning more about our brain.

That summer, I read a scientific article indicating that the various regions of the brain were far more highly interconnected than I had realized. This insight freaked me out. Wait a second, I thought, there are billions of neurons up there in my head talking to each other all the time about *me?* They know more about me than I do? How am I supposed to be in charge? This is *not* fair—my brain is the master, and I am the puppet.

For about a week, I was quite suspicious about my brain and what it was up to. Then I thought, oh well, let's see what we can do about this. Soon enough, I realized that my brain was sitting around up there waiting for work assignments *from me.* My neurons will do the work I give them to do; my brain is more of a servant than a master. That made me feel better. I wanted control, but I settled for influence.

Rebalancing an Underperforming Asset

Intuitively, it seemed logical to take stock of my brain assets in a manner similar to a financial review for clients. Through a self-assessment, I figured out that one of my brain assets, the parietal lobe (associated with physical and hands-on activities), had been the least engaged for the past few years of my life. My parietal lobe was not associated with the strengths that had led me to success in my financial services career or writing. My parietal lobe had become a couch potato. So that looked like the best area to work to heed the advice "use it or lose it."

Engaging this underperforming asset was very difficult. I had to make the time to do things I was not good at and did not like doing, such as dancing and home repairs. Also, something within me—be it habit, a 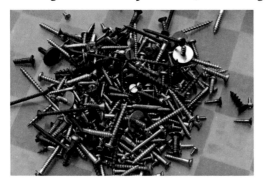 lazy brain, a lack of willpower, identity, gut bacteria, genes, dopamine, or the devil—was resisting my intention, as if using my whole brain to be a whole person was not a deeply compelling goal at some level.

One day, something around the house broke, so I figured it was time to work my parietal lobe and try to fix it myself. While looking for the right type of screw, I tipped over a whole big container with fifty individual compartments, which sent fifty different kinds of nails and screws flying into a pile on the floor.

As I looked at the mess, a thought arose in my mind: "I don't do this. I'll have to get my screw-savvy brother to clean this mess up." Then I said to myself, "Wait a second, who says 'I' don't do this? I say, I do this."

I sorted all the nails and screws back into their little compartments right then and there. It seemed to take forever, and I had no idea what most of them were for, but I had an elated feeling about overcoming the little voice in my mind that had tried to boss me around. This was a turning point for me and my parietal lobe! It had taken me about five years to get there, but it has really paid off, as you'll learn in chapter 6.

My own subsequent success led me to wonder if this "work the least-active brain asset" technique would work for others, too. Inspired by the simple but effective financial pyramid diagram we used in financial services, I developed the Brain Portfolio Tool to help make brain training easier for other people.

In the autumn of 2009, a prototype of the Brain Portfolio Tool was field-tested on a group of fifteen friends, family, and colleagues. This group included men and women ages 30 to 64, most of whom worked full time. I asked them to identify a yearning they had for their lives right now and their least active brain asset. Then they each selected an activity that would work that area and pursued it for four weeks.

The central question this pilot program tested was whether the brain could perform better after deliberately engaging the least active brain asset, motivated by the unfulfilled yearning.

At the end of the four weeks, I asked the participants what they had learned from the program. Here are some of their responses:

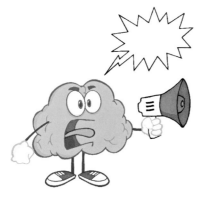

* "The program made me realize that I'm truly resistant to change. . . . I need to become FEARLESS!"

* "I feel much more focused, clear, and passionate about bringing an end to my marriage and moving forward."

* "It has helped me to gain insight into my biggest fear: experiencing pain and suffering. Before I viewed suffering as something to be avoided at all costs; now I see it as part of life that can help me learn and grow. My yearning is to make a difference in people's lives."

* "I learned that my brain is still working OK despite my age. . . . To meet my soulmate I might have to abandon what I was previously focused on, and start afresh, leaving myself open to new possibilities."

- "I know that I will be able to sleep better on those troubled nights by collecting my thoughts and not simply rehearsing them over and over again. I have not found this comfortable in the past, but it seems easier now."

- "Even though we all have strengths and weaknesses and can exercise them, we also need to accept them. It is OK to be me."

- "I have a better chance at remembering aspects of my visual experience than I did before."

- "Early in the program I realized this yearning to reconcile with my daughter. . . . Now I realize that she's the kind of person I have to set serious boundaries with, and due to my personal problems with addiction, this wasn't clear."

In the years following this program, many of these people went on to make major positive changes in their lives, and felt the program helped them along their path. This experiment convinced me that our brain is mobilized by the *consciously articulated* desires of our hearts. However, 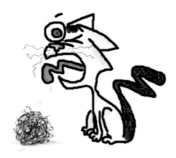 our brain, like a cat, is self-grooming, and chokes on its own activity from time to time and must spit the hairball out to resume normal operations (integration). As we get older, our brain will function best if we cough up the emotional "hairballs" of our younger years.

Since this pilot program, the Brain Portfolio Tool has been renamed, reworked, and introduced to hundreds of people of all ages, many of whom have also found it beneficial. It's not the only way to manage your brain assets; you may find other approaches that work for you. But make sure you see our brain for what it is: the most valuable asset in the universe.

Brain wealth Billionaires

Most people think of our brain as a depreciating asset, but as we learned in the introduction, neuroscientists have reversed this opinion within the past thirty years. After the age of thirty, our brain deliberately begins to sacrifice speed and efficiency for the sake of integration and wisdom. If we measure by the appropriate benchmarks, the older brain is a better brain. (If this sounds redundant, good. The brainwashing has worked, and you have now fully absorbed this important truth.)

To get started with the Brain Portfolio Tool, we need to adopt the mindset of a very rich investor. We can liken our brain's 100 billion neurons to a $100 billion portfolio that needs to be diversified and managed in order to appreciate. When it comes to brain wealth, we are all billionaires!

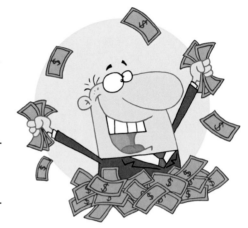

It's been said that compound interest is the eighth wonder of the world. Neuroplasticity, the capacity to keep building a wealth of new neural connections, is our brain's equivalent of compound interest. Though the average adult brain has about 500 trillion neural connections, it's possible to double this number—and no, it won't require a bigger skull to accommodate this growth. Conversely, if we let our brain do the equivalent of hiding its wealth under the mattress by failing to engage in life, our brain assets can lose value.

The aim of brain training with the Brain Portfolio Tool is to increase your brain wealth—*and our species' collective brain wealth*—by expanding your capabilities as a human being. The idea is not to be a perfect person, but a balanced, whole person as you advance in the direction of your hopes and dreams.

Brain training must be used for a personally meaningful outcome to achieve success. If you don't have a yearning way down deep inside, your brain knows it, and it won't waste its efforts. Similarly, if you don't believe you can do something, your thrifty brain knows and won't waste its efforts, because it knows the negative belief will hamper neuroplasticity: mind over gray matter.

But what if you badly want to achieve something, yet lack the confidence to push forward to your goal? The influence of someone else who believes in you can fill your mind with confidence the way a pump fills a flat tire with air. For example, the teacher Annie Sullivan helped Helen Keller to learn language even though she was blind, deaf, and mute. She went on to become the first deafblind person to earn a bachelor of arts degree. She worked as an author, political activist, and lecturer and lived until the age 87.

In case you do not have your own personal Annie Sullivan, I want you to know that I believe in you. If you are absorbing these words right now, you are capable of doing anything with our brain that you yearn for, regardless of your age, degrees, financial wealth, gender, hair color, income, marital status, nationality, occupation, political affiliation, race, religion, sexual orientation, or any other superficial labels that apply to you. You are a member of our species, and you share the human brain—that's all you need.

> Alone we can do so little.
> Together we can do so much.
> HELEN KELLER

Remember Gabrielle Giffords' story, and how hard she worked for a year just to move her right hand. And remember Albert and Robert from chapter 3, who each had only half a brain yet led rewarding lives. You have a huge store of brain wealth to work with. Think of all you can do with it!

So think of yourself as a brain-wealth investor with a huge pool of assets that can easily gain or lose value, and let's get started.

Brain Portfolio Tool Overview

The main value of the Brain Portfolio Tool is that it shows how our various brain assets relate to key aspects of daily living, including our mental range of motion as well as activities at home or work. By using this tool to assess how fully we invest in (or use) each type of brain asset, we can formulate a plan for growing our brain wealth.

The Brain Portfolio Tool is presented in figures 4.1, 4.2, and 4.3, and in the worksheet at the end of this chapter. In figure 4.1, titled "The Brain Portfolio Tool: Brain Asset Attributes," the top half of the first illustration shows a color-coded map of our brain assets. To highlight the most important aspects of the brain, the illustration has been simplified as follows:

✳ Only the left hemisphere is shown; however, the same components of the brain are present in the right hemisphere as well.

✳ The default network (the line in red) is shown on the outside of the cerebral cortex, even though most of its activity takes place along the inside (medial) surfaces of our left and right hemispheres.

Below the brain diagram, a table indicates the mental range of motion, outlook, focus, and muse associated with each brain asset.

Figure 4.2 is on the facing page, titled "The Brain Portfolio Tool: Brain Asset Returns." This diagram contains a model of a brain portfolio with five color-coded sections to correspond to the brain assets in the first diagram. The most important feature of the image is the anchoring of brain assets around the self and the default network. In addition, two key attributes are indicated for each of the five categories:

1. Key cultural tool supported by each brain asset

2. Key human value supported by each brain asset

Below the brain portfolio diagram, a table indicates the returns on investment that occur when a brain asset has low returns (too little activity, underinvested), high returns (an ideal level of activity, target allocation), or negative returns (too much activity, overinvested).

The purpose of this highly simplified table is to help you identify brain assets that are underinvested. If you look at this table and determine that you have negative returns on a brain asset, don't feel too bad. You're not alone. I have met only two people who felt they had a well-balanced brain portfolio—both women in their nineties who were in excellent cognitive health.

It is very difficult to reduce activity in an overinvested brain asset. The best approach is to focus on increasing activity in an underinvested brain asset and let the brain figure out how to rebalance the activity of the various assets.

Brain Asset Attributes

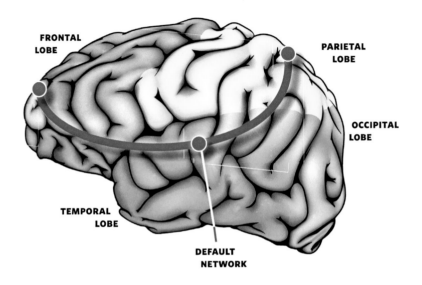

BRAIN ASSET	RANGE OF MOTION	OUTLOOK	FOCUS	MUSE
Parietal	Adventure	Courageous	The unknown	Objects
Occipital	Achievement	Organized	The score	Images
Temporal	Attachment	Trusting	The heart	People
Frontal	Adaptation	Hopeful	The future	Ideas
Default network	Autobiography	Empathetic	The self	Stories

Figure 4.1. The Brain Portfolio Tool: Brain Asset Attributes

Brain Asset Returns

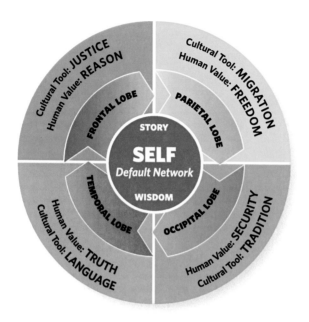

BRAIN ASSET	LOW RETURNS (underinvested)	HIGH RETURNS (target allocation)	NEGATIVE RETURNS (overinvested)
Parietal	Reactive	Spontaneous	Wild
Occipital	Careless	Conscientious	Controlling
Temporal	Detached	Compassionate	Obsessed
Frontal	Distracted	Visionary	Arrogant
Default network	Shallow	Authentic	Isolated

Figure 4.2. The Brain Portfolio Tool: Brain Asset Returns

THE BRAIN PORTFOLIO TOOL

Activities by Brain Asset

PARIETAL LOBE

Bicycle/motorcyle riding*
Building objects or structures*
Camping*
Crafts*
Dancing*
Drawing*
Driving*
Gym workout or classes*
Hands-on work*
Hiking*
Horseback riding*
Hunting*
Knitting, sewing*
Outdoor adventures*
Performing magic tricks*
Repairs and maintenance*
Sculpture*
Sports*
Survival skills*
Swimming*
Tennis*
Use of equipment and objects*
Woodworking*

OCCIPITAL LOBE

Administrative activity*
Art*
Attending/watching sporting events
Attending banquets
Committee work
Competitive tournaments*
Computer work
Design-fashion, games, movies*
Gambling
Games of chance: board games, cards, video games
Household maintenance routines*
Instruction*
Movies
Museums
Paperwork*
Photography*
Policies and procedures
Political skills*
Rules and regulations
Teamwork*
Travel (cruises or familiar places)*

Figure 4.3. The Brain Portfolio Tool: Activities by Brain Asset

**Significant motor output required by the brain.*

TEMPORAL LOBE

Acting*

Art of conversation*

Cooking for family and friends*

Diplomatic skills*

Gardening*

Helping others

Improvisation*

Inclusion/diversity activity*

Journaling*

Language/learning a new language*

Listening

Mentoring*

Music: listening, playing instrument*

Play reading group*

Preaching*

Nursing, caregiving*

Relationship skills*

Remembering faces and names

Scrapbooking/genealogy*

Singing*

Social justice advocacy*

Spiritual/personal growth

Storytelling*

Support groups*

Teaching*

Tending relationships*

Volunteering to help others*

Writing*

FRONTAL LOBE

Astronomy

Attending lectures (listening)

Bridge

Chess

Critical thinking skills

Decision-making skills

Discussion groups*

Emotional management (self-talk)

Envisioning the future

Financial planning*

Golf*

Leadership skills*

Logical analysis

Long-term planning

Math

Mind training: meditation, mindfulness,
    tai chi*, yoga*

Public speaking*

Setting and achieving goals*

Speech*

Strategy

Travel (unfamiliar places)*

DEFAULT NETWORK

Assessing intentions and motives

Autobiographical writing*

Daydreaming

Developing one's personal story

Empathy

Humor: detecting, using

Identifying personal passion and
    purpose

Imagining one's personal future

Learning from past experiences

Listening to stories

Personal reflection on ethics, feelings

Reading fiction

Reading plays

Reminiscing, nostalgia

Serving needs of others

Taking a third-party perspective on
    self/others

Taking charge of one's abilities
    and goals

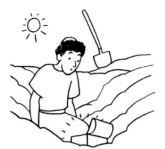 Think of underinvested assets as buried treasure rather than weaknesses. They represent excellent opportunities for growth and further investment. By boosting activity in your least-invested asset, you will help your whole brain become stronger, more efficient, and better integrated.

Figure 4.3 indicates some of the activities that engage each of the five brain assets. Note the following general parameters:

1. *Brain assets act as leaders.* No activity on the list engages only one brain asset. However, different activities require leadership by different brain assets, recruiting other brain assets to get the job done. It's important that each brain asset has a chance to exercise leadership, particularly after age 40, to facilitate brain integration and avoid cognitive inflexibility. So this is a simplified approach to help us connect brain-asset leadership to everyday activities. For example, watching a movie is primarily a visual activity, so "Movies" is listed in the occipital (green) category. Listening to music is primarily an auditory activity, so it is listed under the temporal (pink) category.

2. *The front of the brain needs the most exercise after age 30.* Leisure activities such as art, chess, singing, or writing are hard work for our brain, since they require leadership by less efficient brain assets (temporal, frontal, default network). Activities such as performing tasks on a computer or gadget, physical exercise, reading, or watching a movie do not work the brain as hard, as they call more on highly efficient brain asset leaders toward the back of the brain (the occipital and parietal lobes). As we grow older, the need to "use it or lose it" requires increasing engagement of the least efficient brain assets.

3. *Asterisks indicate output.* Our brain is like our gastrointestinal tract: too much input and not enough output causes constipation. The brain areas dedicated to sensory input and motor output are highly efficient. The vast majority of our brain's cerebral cortex is composed of association cortex areas, which process incoming information for

one primary purpose: to help the frontal lobe plan and execute adaptive, goal-directed, self-determined behavior in any given situation. There are three forms of motor activity executed by the frontal lobe: movement of the whole body; movement of the limbs; and speech. So the term *motor mouth* for someone who talks excessively is scientifically accurate. Movement of the body and limbs works both sides of the brain, while speech is primarily a left-brain activity.

4. *Cognitive flexibility is not optional.* Cognitive inflexibility, a suspected risk factor for Alzheimer's, can arise from excessive engagement of one or two brain assets or one hemisphere after age 40. Using the brain assets associated with our strengths works well at younger ages, but in middle age our brain switches gears, working to integrate the activity of all brain assets, not just the strongest ones. Excessive reliance on one or two brain assets for decades may lead to burnout and impede integration. The ultimate goal is whole-brain engagement, which gives us cognitive flexibility and a full range of mental motion.

Brain Asset Self-Assessment

It's time to roll up your sleeves and get to work in assessing your own brain asset activity. We'll work through the Brain Portfolio Worksheet at the end of the chapter step by step to identify any brain assets that may be underinvested (under-invested, not un-invested). Don't worry about precise estimates; a ballpark estimate is all that is needed. If you don't want to take the time to go through these steps, you can cut to the chase by looking at the table of returns in figure 4.2 and identifying your least-invested brain asset.

STEP ONE: **Indicate the most important yearning you have right now.** Indicate something that you truly long for in your life. This could involve your love life, family, friends, health, lifestyle, work, community, or purpose in life, but it needs to have a personal connection to you rather than being too general, such as peace on earth.

STEP TWO: **Describe your current activities in each brain asset category below.** Refer to figure 4.3 to figure out what brain assets you're using the most in your current lifestyle. Generally, the type of sensory input is the determining factor of which brain asset is acting as leader. The occipital, parietal, and temporal lobes are engaged primarily by their respective sensory inputs. The frontal lobe and default network are engaged with mental activity generated by the sensory information received from the occipital, parietal, and temporal lobes. To account for activities that don't occur daily, consider looking at your activities over a typical week or month.

STEP THREE: Indicate in the right margin the percentage of time given to each brain asset. Again, precision is not required. Try to figure out what brain assets are engaged in the activities you spend the most time with. For example, if you spend eight hours a day in front of a screen (computer, tablet, phone, television, or movie) for seven days a week, the occipital lobe (brain asset leader for visual activity) would account for 50 percent of your weekly activity. A week has 168 hours (7 days × 24 hours), with about 112 hours left after sleeping and personal care. This much screen time adds up to 56 hours (8 hours a day × 7 days a week), which is half of 112 hours.

STEP FOUR: Rank your brain assets by amount of activity. Based on the estimates in step 2, rank the brain assets from most active (1) to least active (5). Indicate the rank on the line to the left of each brain asset.

STEP FIVE: Underline the brain asset that is most engaged in your daily life. Underline the brain asset that is ranked number 1. This is your most active asset.

STEP SIX: Circle the brain asset that is least engaged in your daily life. Circle the brain asset that is ranked number 5. This is your least active asset.

If at all possible, discuss your self-assessment with a small group of trusted friends and ask them for input. It is impossible to get an accurate picture of yourself from your perspective alone. People you trust will be able to help identify both your mental strengths and your challenges. If two or more other people say the same thing about you, they are probably right. But you are the final arbiter of anything to do with you and your brain.

Now that you have completed the self-assessment, you are ready to tap neuroplasticity to expand your capabilities. When it comes to brain wealth, we generate profits through learning. Whatever the brain asset you are working on, the process is the same: learn something new that will encourage the brain to grow new connections (profit) in that area.

Once you have selected an underinvested brain asset to work, choose an activity that will "invest" in that asset. Figure 4.3 provides a list of suggested activities that can be used to develop each brain asset. Consult the brain asset descriptions in chapter 3 to get ideas for other activities that might be appropriate for your goals.

Do the specified activity for at least fifteen minutes a day for at least four weeks to get the brain investing in new synaptic connections. Be patient and focus on the process: the goal is to build new connections, not to master the new activity right away.

Remember, you are trying to influence the most complex structure in the universe! The older you are, the longer it may take to see results, as our brain has more wealth (connections) to keep track of as we get older.

If you encounter too much inner resistance, reach out to someone for help or encouragement. Better yet, take a class. As we learned from chapter 2, our brain hates to become too isolated. Social activity of some sort may provide the jolt of oxytocin your brain needs to learn something new quickly. Or pick a different brain asset to work.

The engagement questions were intentionally omitted in this chapter, since the Brain Portfolio Tool self-assessment includes engagement topics. In chapter 5, we'll learn some brain training tips and tricks from other people to help you get results quickly.

It matters not how strait the gate,
How charged with punishments the scroll,
I am the master of my fate,
I am the captain of my soul.

WILLIAM ERNEST HENLEY, *Invictus*

---

worksheet

1. Indicate the most important yearning you have right now.

2. Describe your current activities in each brain asset category below.

3. Indicate in the right margin the percentage of time given to each brain asset.

4. Rank the brain assets listed below from 1 to 5 (1 is most active) on the lines to the left of the asset names.

5. Underline the brain asset that is most engaged in your daily life.

6. Circle the brain asset that is least engaged in your daily life.

YEARNING:

_____

_____   ▢ **PARIETAL LOBE** _____

_____

_____   ▢ **OCCIPITAL LOBE** _____

_____

_____   ▢ **TEMPORAL LOBE** _____

_____

_____   ▢ **FRONTAL LOBE** _____

_____

_____   ▢ **DEFAULT NETWORK** _____

_____

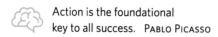

CHAPTER 5 Tips for Growing Brain Assets

Action is the foundational
key to all success. PABLO PICASSO

L et's stop and look at the ground we have covered so far. We've
learned about our brain's back story and about how neuroplasticity
is the key to getting better with age. We've become acquainted with our
five brain assets and the mental range of motion they deliver:

* Parietal lobe: Adventure

* Occipital lobe: Achievement

* Temporal lobe: Attachment

* Frontal lobe: Adaptation

* Default network: Autobiography

We have also explored how to use the Brain Portfolio Tool to manage
our brain like a portfolio of appreciating assets to get better with age.
And now, the million-dollar question before us is this:

How can I tell if my brain wealth is growing?

The answer to this question is easy: if you're learning, it's growing.
Anything we learn, from the name of someone we just met to a new skill
or habit, requires our brain to grow new synaptic connections.

You cannot recall anything you have not learned, and you can't learn
anything without paying attention. Attention is guided by intention, and
intention is driven by yearnings, which grow out of the soil of meaningful life experiences.

In other words, our brain is not going to go through the hard work
of building new connections unless it's for something we really want
way down deep inside: a yearning. Our brain *will* do the heavy lifting of
building new connections for something that is meaningful in the context of our identity, relationships, and culture.

75

When we wonder if our efforts are producing any results, it's natural to compare ourselves to others. In financial services, one of the first questions a new client would ask me was, "How does my net worth compare to that of others like me?" So I can imagine that some readers may be wondering how their brain assets stack up.

The answer, though, is that there's no quantitative measure of brain assets. All attempts to benchmark the performance of human brains have failed to capture the essence of being human. For example, grades in school, standardized test scores, IQ tests, brain volume, advanced degrees, salary, and personal wealth are not reliable indicators of brain wealth—or of a life well lived by a member of the human species, for that matter.

This lack of correlation between extrinsic measures and successful living is due in part to our brain's variability. Our brains are like fingerprints: they share the same structures, but no two people's are identical. Also, our brain assets carry the inner movements of the life force within us—emotions, feelings, thoughts, memories, beliefs, values—that exert tremendous influence over our life choices but are difficult to pin down, let alone measure.

We don't know Mother Nature's benchmarks for evaluating our brain assets. She has given us so much *freedom* with the most complex structure in the universe! Yet clearly there are a set of warranty conditions that we need to abide by to ensure cognitive health and get better with age. Three conditions we can safely assume are the needs for social connection, lifelong learning, and neuroplasticity. Neuroplasticity and the mandate to "use it or lose it" are the keys to getting better with age.

The growth of new synaptic connections can best be assessed by the evidence of these outcomes:

1. Learning new behavior, information, skills, or ways of thinking

2. The execution of new forms of output (action, behavior, or speech)

3. A personally satisfying gain or success

4. A noticeable improvement in cognitive function, such as memory

However, age and culture have a significant influence on neuroplasticity. Is it easier to grow new connections at younger ages? You betcha. Is it easier to grow new connections for behaviors encouraged by your social context? You betcha. Is it easier to grow new connections that flow from your identity? You betcha. Are there some tips for growing brain assets at different ages? You betcha.

But if I just tell you what these tips are, you won't absorb the information, because they are so simple. So I'll tell you in a way that will help you remember, through the stories of six people from different generations. All of these tips can be useful at any age, not just at the age indicated in the example.

Billy: From Brat to Brilliant (Internet Generation)

As a volunteer in our local Desert Reach Program, I am part of a team that goes to fourth-grade classrooms to teach kids about the Sonoran Desert with hands-on activities. A couple of years ago, I showed up in a classroom and was surprised to see a smiling, familiar face: Billy, the ten-year-old son of an associate named Kate.*

During the ninety-minute program, I observed how Billy behaved—or, rather, misbehaved. I could tell he was very bright, but he was out of control relative to the other ten-year-old boys in the class. When his mother heard I had been there and asked how Billy was in class, I said he was obviously bright and omitted the rest of the story. She was a single parent over age 50; I knew she was trying her best with him. And I'm not a parent, so what do I know?

A few weeks later, Kate told me she was concerned about an upcoming conference with Billy's teacher. Billy's grades were dropping, and she was convinced it was because the teacher was being too hard on him.

I told her that the teacher seemed impressive compared to the other fourth-grade teachers I had met. Then I asked what the teacher said about how Billy was acting in class. She reported that the teacher

---

* Throughout this chapter, all names and some narrative details have been changed to respect the privacy of these individuals.

said he didn't listen and was disruptive and disrespectful to other kids. I said, "That's how he was when I was there." She was appalled and wanted more details.

I told her my impression was that he struggled with emotional regulation, and she said "Huh?" I said he lacked impulse control, and she responded that he was a ten-year-old boy. But she accepted my observation that the other boys in the class were able to restrain themselves better and acknowledged that this was an important life skill for him to acquire if he wanted to go to college one day.

When she asked me what she could do to help Billy, my suggestion was to get him to play chess. I had heard at a neuroscience conference for educators that chess was successfully being used as an intervention for attention deficit–hyperactivity disorder in kids because it built connections in the left frontal lobe, the brain area responsible for executive functions such as emotional management and impulse control.

The school year was almost over. I suggested that Kate start Billy on playing chess over the summer. Given how easy it is for a young brain to build new connections, he could have a new and improved brain by the

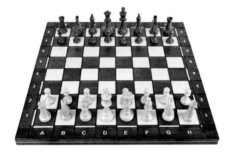

time he returned to school in August.

A couple of weeks later, Kate said she was learning chess with Billy. A couple of weeks after that, she said while Billy liked chess, she hated it, so she had made a deal with a family friend to play chess with Billy while she cooked dinner for both of them. Not surprisingly, Billy enjoyed the attention from a friendly adult and learned quickly.

When Billy returned to school that August, he started getting straight A's and behaving in class. He doesn't play much chess anymore, but his success as a student, Boy Scout, athlete, and all-round person has continued.

Through playing chess, Billy grew some new synaptic connections in his frontal lobe that delivered a greater range of motion for *adaptation* to the social challenges he faced at school. By playing with a nurturing male family friend, Billy also grew some new connections in the temporal lobe, enabling a deeper level of *attachment*. For children under age 12, achievement follows attachment.

Billy's success demonstrates how our brain is born to learn throughout life *within a social context*. Anyone can train our brain to improve *at any age* if they choose to and work at it, as Billy did—and can continue to do so even into their nineties, as Pablo Picasso did—as long as the learning is rooted in the social soil.

Our brain learns best when trust exceeds anxiety. When it feels safe, it knows it has the leeway to spend time building new connections rather than coping with imminent threats.

TIP #1: Seeds of learning sprout best when rooted in supportive social soil.

Jeffrey: Tell Me about This Brain Stuff (Millennial Generation)

A couple of years ago, I got a call from Jeffrey, the nineteen-year-old son of a good friend. He said, "I want to hear about this brain stuff you are doing." I was astonished, as no teenager I knew had ever seemed particularly curious about our brain.

At the time, Jeffrey was a student at a local community college, developing a career as a musician, and living at home. We had known him for many years and had enjoyed hearing him play jazz music with other students over the years, at gigs that paid him little or no money.

We scheduled a time to get together for a brain portfolio review. I waived the usual fee, since he was not earning much; and I figured it would be good market research, as I had never worked with someone in this age group before.

When we got together, I asked him what he was hoping to get out of our time together. He said he was doing well at school and filled me in on the various girls he had been dating (not that I had asked). His career as a musician was also going well. However, a teacher had asked him to play with a professional band at a fundraiser for the school, and he felt it was taking him too long to learn a new song, compared to the other musicians. He wondered if his brain could learn faster to help him keep up.

I affirmed his curiosity, and then asked if he was nervous about stepping up to play in a bigger league. He said, "Maybe." We discussed the role of anxiety in learning: sometimes it can be helpful, pushing the brain to do its best, but too much anxiety interferes with the brain's ability to learn.

We reviewed the Brain Portfolio Tool, and he identified the parietal brain asset, associated with adventure and risk taking, as his least active area.

Many of the recommended activities for developing connections in the parietal lobe involve physical exercise or hands-on activity. He was not currently doing any physical activity and objected to the idea of 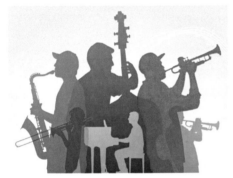 going to the gym. I assured him that the choice was his, but if he wanted his brain to perform better, he might benefit from working this under-invested area, since it helps boost working memory and learning.

When I asked if there was another parietal-boosting activity that interested him, he looked at the Brain Portfolio Tool and mentioned running, which he used to do on the track team in high school. He decided to start running again.

The next month, his mom and I attended the fundraiser. Jeffrey had two solos, a sign of the band's confidence in him. He was phenomenal! He was also thrilled to have us there in the audience. As we left, I said to my friend, "Jeffrey has grown up."

In the months that followed, he scaled new heights. He formed a new band under his own name, with one of his teachers playing in it! We attended a major jazz festival that featured Jeffrey and his band, a gig that not only gained him recognition but also paid decently. He also became more adventurous: when he received a scholarship to a four-year college, he accepted it, even though it meant moving to another state where he had no contacts. He even talked about getting a motorcycle, but, fortunately for his mother's peace of mind, he hasn't followed through on that idea yet.

The effect of physical exercise on our brain is a widely researched topic. As we learned in chapter 3, all physical movement requires both hemispheres to work together, which can help regulate emotional activity. While exercise alone cannot guarantee brain health, it has been shown to reduce anxiety and therefore may help protect neurons from toxic chemicals released by stress. Moreover, some neurotropic growth factors that encourage neuroplasticity are stored in the fingers and toes and are released through physical exercise.

TIP #2: Physical exercise can reduce toxic anxiety, enable learning, and build confidence.

Richard: Taking care of Everyone but Me (Generation X)

When I began my career as a brain coach in 2007, a thirty-eight-year-old financial services sales colleague named Richard contacted me for an appointment. We met soon thereafter, and I asked him what was going on. He was upset about the impending divorce of another colleague in the office, whose wife was leaving him. Richard's circumstances were similar to this individual's, with a wife at home with little kids. Richard didn't think divorce could happen to him, but he hadn't thought it could happen to the other guy, either. Richard told me that if he lost his family, it would ruin his life.

As we spoke, he shared the conflicts he felt. While at work, he felt guilty about not spending time with his family, and while with his family, he felt he should be working to make more money. The family's finances were okay, but his wife wanted a bigger home, and he dreaded the thought of higher monthly expenses.

As a result of these conflicts, his health and mood were suffering. When he was at home, he worked in his study and yelled at the kids if they interrupted him. He didn't sleep well at night. If he were his wife, he said, he wouldn't want to be married to someone like him.

After he blurted all this out, I said, "Richard, I am a brain coach. You need a therapist." He said he had already tried therapy and medications, but they hadn't worked, and he was wondering if some kind of brain training could help. I said I had no idea if it could help with all that, but we could try.

We reviewed the Brain Portfolio Tool. I asked him to make a check-mark next to the activities he did outside work. He looked at the list and said, "I don't do any of this." Then we considered how he used his brain assets at work, and Richard determined that the parietal asset was his least active area. He reflected that he used to go to the gym but had stopped to make more time for work, and then he had gained weight.

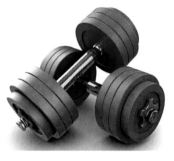

I suggested that he find some way to engage his parietal lobe when he wasn't working to re-balance his brain assets.

A few months later, I checked in to see how things were going. Richard said he had started going to the gym again, putting it into his calendar as if it were a client appointment. He had joined a "Biggest Loser" program and lost twenty pounds. Every week, he made a little time to be by himself and do something he wanted to do.

In hindsight, Richard thought our brain portfolio review meeting had helped him realize his life was out of balance. He said, "I was so worried about taking care of my family and my clients, I forgot about taking care of myself. But if I don't take care of myself, I can't take care of them." By taking better care of himself, he became more self-aware and was able to improve both his relationships and productivity.

Over the next few years, he made some changes at work to decrease his stress level and increase his productivity. When real estate prices tanked, Richard and his family found a great deal on a property that gave them more elbow room and more opportunities for active family time outdoors. Despite the economic downturn, he had his best year ever and wasn't worried about the additional expense of buying the new home.

He was even able to start thinking about what else he might want to do with his life once his kids were grown.

After five years, he reflected on the brain portfolio review and said, "This information helped me sort through some challenges and take my sales production to a whole new level without sacrificing my personal quality of life."

Richard had experienced the work-life balance crisis that typically arises at the end of Stage 2. By rebalancing his brain assets, Richard made a successful mid-life transition to Stage 3.

TIP #3: Taking care of yourself can help you resolve inner conflicts and improve important relationships at home and work.

---

carol: Have I Become Stupid?
(Baby Boomer)

Carol, a fifty-two-year-old information technology manager with an Ivy League education, was worried about losing her job. After attending one of my "Brain Investors" programs, she sent me this note:

> I gotta tell you: your talk really shook something loose in me. I was struck by your saying that when someone is hostile to something, their brain totally shuts down from learning it. I am definitely hostile to the new software program that I have to learn to do my job. And I have such a hard time learning it that I once asked my husband to tell me in all honesty whether he thinks I've become really stupid. He said no, but I really can't know if that was honesty or tact, can I? Anyway, in pondering this I felt little flashes of accep-
> tance and interest in my job. The 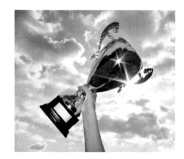 winds changed with this accep-
> tance. I was able to learn and apply the new program success-fully. Instead of getting fired from my job, I got a "Most Valu-able Employee" award. I was

absolutely shocked. Thanks for saying things that catalyzed my growth.

At age 52, Carol needed to align her goal with her inner *autobiographical self,* orchestrated by her default network brain asset. With regard to the learning challenge she faced at work, her initial answer to the question "Who am I?" was "I am not someone who needs to learn this new software program." Once her identity changed to incorporate the goal ("I am someone who *wants* to learn this new software program"), she got quick and excellent results.

As Carol discovered, our brainpower is best accessed through **intrinsic motivation**, an inner desire to seek out new experiences and challenges as we build out the blueprint of our lives in personally meaningful ways.

Conversely, **extrinsic motivation** underlies behavior that is driven by external rewards such as money, fame, social status, grades, praise, compliance, or other forms of social recognition. Extrinsic motivation arises from outside the individual, while intrinsic motivation originates inside the individual.

Identity alignment and intrinsic motivation are especially important to change long-term behavior related to diet, exercise, smoking, and substance abuse.

TIP #4: Align identity with a goal to tap intrinsic motivation and make learning easier, especially over age 40.

George: I Have Had Cognitive Improvement (The Silent Generation)

Life is like investing: you cannot avoid losses, but if you offset them with gains, you end up ahead. When teaching, I remind people to focus on their next gain, rather than what they have lost, to boost brain health and cognitive function.

In the retirement communities where I teach, some people seem fixated on the losses they have experienced in life. A refreshing exception was a man named George. At the beginning of class one day, I asked who had been doing something to work their brain, as I usually do. George raised his hand and said, "I want to share with everyone that I have had significant cognitive improvement." He cited recovery of functionality in the areas of balance, speech, and focus.

His peers wanted to know what he did to get these results. He mentioned the medications that he was taking, which suggested he had been diagnosed with Alzheimer's. But he attributed his improvement to new habits: going to the gym every day, taking some new classes, and staying away from the computer and television.

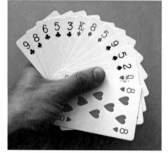

Someone else in our class said they had recently noticed a big improvement in how George played bridge. Everyone was impressed by his resolve! I was amazed at his frankness and willingness to trust the people around him.

Many people seem to fold their cards when they get a diagnosis of mild cognitive impairment or Alzheimer's. George shows us how resilient the brain can be if we apply the power of positive thinking to our own selves.

TIP #5: Don't let a diagnosis get you down: pursue neuroplasticity with vigor.

Gloria: she'll get me going (the GI Generation)

As part of a Brain Awareness Week celebration several years ago, I was conducting brain portfolio reviews during a wellness fair at a retirement community where I teach. Independent living residents signed up for individual appointments. One resident, Gloria, was a gracious, smiling woman with a pleasant Southern accent.

I asked Gloria if she had a goal in mind for our appointment, and she indicated that she was mostly just curious about what I did. We reviewed the Brain Portfolio Tool, discussed the benefits of rebalancing the brain portfolio, and identified retirement-community activities that offered "investment opportunities" in the different brain assets.

Gloria looked at all the activities and said in her Southern drawl, "My, my, all this is available? I'm not doing anything. My husband died, and I have had some health problems, but now I better get busy." She identified the brain asset which was the most underinvested and chose a class that would increase her investment in that brain asset.

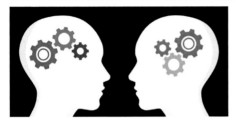

When asked how she would overcome the adult brain's innate resistance to shifting gears, Gloria thought for a few seconds and then responded, "I'll call Mary, a friend of mine who is in that class: she'll get me going." Gloria's mental agility and social instincts were so impressive that I asked her if she would mind telling me her age. She smiled warmly and said, "Ninety-three."

TIP #6: Find a brain buddy who can help you overcome cognitive change resistance.

Always bear in mind that your own resolution to succeed
is more important than any other.
ABRAHAM LINCOLN

Engagement Questions

1. Which of the six stories can you relate to the most? Why?

2. Which of the six tips do you find the most helpful and why? Are there any you would add?

3. Which of these cognitive activities do you find most challenging to engage and why: learning, memory, attention, intention?

4. Is it difficult or easy for you to understand the desires of your heart and tap your inner motivation? Why? Is there someone you know who is good at this? What tricks do they use to channel intrinsic motivation?

5. How do you think you are doing in following the advice "use it or lose it"?

6. What new capabilities or skills that you've learned in the past few years are you especially proud of?

7. Who is your brain buddy? If you don't have one, who can you ask to be your partner in this way?

CHAPTER 6 **Honing the superpowers**

Life can only be understood backwards; but it must be lived forwards.
SØREN KIERKEGAARD

How happy I would be if you were not even reading this chapter—if you had already put this book down and embarked on your own personal learning adventure to buff up your neurons so you and your brain can get better with age. How happy I would be if you had already evaluated your brain portfolio, selected a brain asset to work on, chosen the activity you planned to do, determined where and when to take a class, figured out how to fit the class into your schedule and budget, developed a plan to overcome your inertia, and started on building new synaptic connections right where you need them: in your least active brain asset.

But if you're still reading, we may as well address the all-important subject of implementation. Making changes—little ones or big ones—to behavior, beliefs, and identity is where the rubber meets the road in brain training. As Stephen Sondheim put it in *Sunday in the Park with George*, "Having just a vision's no solution, everything depends on execution."

In my teaching about neuroplasticity and the Brain Portfolio Tool, many people have said to me, "I know what I should do, but I have trouble following through." Surprisingly, some people in their eighties and nineties have been more effective at changing their behavior than people half their age, even in the wake of a significant loss. Such people have good access to special capacities that we have not yet discussed in any detail.

It takes energy, or vitality, to overcome inertia and make desired changes in thoughts, words, or deeds. Commonly referred to as mojo, vitality is defined as a lively or energetic quality that conveys the power to survive and thrive. As the Latin root *vita* (life) suggests, vitality comes from the life force itself; it is the antidote to entropy (dissipation of energy).

When it comes to vitality, our brain provides the keys to the kingdom, granting access to special powers unique to our species. So just in case you need them at some point in your brain training adventures, we will now get to know these special powers and see how they help us to get better with age.

Defining the superpowers

For decades, researchers have been trying to understand how brain activity correlates to mental activity in both healthy and impaired people. While many questions remain unanswered, some recent advances have led to a basic understanding of the three major mental modes that we experience during our waking hours, presented here in order of early development:

Executive Functions (EF): a set of abilities that direct nonroutinized behavior for self-determined goals. EF gives us the brain reins to steer our own behavior toward desirable outcomes and get things done in the world.

Sensory-Motor Functions (SM): a set of abilities for experiencing embodiment, emotions, and interpersonal relationships. SM enables us to be aware of the environment and people around us, as well as our body's internal physiological regulation responses such as respiration, hunger, heart rate, and temperature.

Theory of Mind (ToM): a set of abilities for understanding the mental states—the beliefs, desires, feelings, intentions, motivations, and perspectives—of other people, and for realizing how their mental states are different from our own. ToM allows us to develop *narratives* to understand and predict the behavior of self and others.

Let me take a moment to say that it makes me deeply sad, dear reader, to be writing about our most advanced behavioral abilities in this way. The jargon used by scientists to describe EF, SM, and ToM fails to capture the mystery and magic of the human experience. What makes me especially sad is that I can't find the right words to make EF, SM, and ToM sound as exciting to you as they are to me.

As any three-year-old knows, what makes us human should stir the soul and quicken the pulse over and over again every day! Yet the opposite often happens: we take our EF, SM, and ToM for granted until we lose them. I hear Joni Mitchell's voice singing, "Don't it always seem to go, that you don't know what you've got till it's gone."

Many of the neurological malfunctions that are household words today interfere with EF, SM, and ToM, so these abilities are often understood better by their absence than their presence. The gradual loss of voluntary movement wrought by Parkinson's disease, for example, reveals the essence of EF. A fading ability to remember the faces and names of loved ones shows how Alzheimer's interferes with ToM. The loneliness of depression illustrates the loss of SM.

To enliven our exploration of this subject, I am going to refer to EF, ToM, and SM as our *superpowers,* because this term captures their true nature better than the jargon does. Although we may refer to these three superpowers separately, they are inseparable in brain, mind, and DNA. Figure 6.1 illustrates how our brain juggles the three superpowers to produce behavior.

Now let's take a closer look at how our unique human superpowers relate to daily life:

Self Superpower (SM): the power to relate. Physical, emotional, and social in nature, the Self Superpower yearns for loving relationships that make the universe a safe, friendly place (figure 6.1, bottom).

Story Superpower (ToM): the power to narrate. Emotional, social, and rational in nature, the Story Superpower knits our personal experiences together into a coherent life story that can be shared with others (figure 6.1, top right).

Steer Superpower (EF): the power to serve. Rationally and socially inclined, our Steer Superpower (figure 6.1, top left) directs cognitive resources to manage emotions and execute marching orders from the

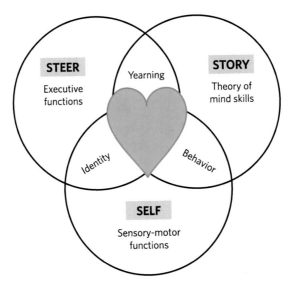

Figure 6.1. Anchored by the heart, our superpowers work together to generate our personal experience of life.

heart (figure 6.1, bottom center), the nexus of our Self and Story Superpowers. This superpower is supported by the machinery of culture: constant teaching and learning.

Back in chapter 2, we learned about the three major networks that the brain aims to develop and integrate over the human life span: sensory-motor; cognitive control; and default mode. See figure 2.4 for a refresher on which brain areas are involved in these three networks.

As figure 6.1 indicates, these three networks also support our superpowers. Self is associated with sensory-motor functions, Story is associated with theory of mind skills and the default network, while Steer is associated with executive functions and the cognitive control network. The heart is the nexus of our superpowers, from cradle to grave.

The neurological foundation for our superpowers is established in lower, subcortical brain regions by ages 3–5, followed by the development of higher cortical regions. These brain areas continue to grow throughout life by means of neuroplasticity, allowing our superpowers to strengthen and get better with age, yielding a powerful inner state described by Mahatma Gandhi as "soul force."

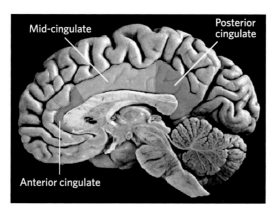

Figure 6.2. The cingulate cortex, part of the primitive limbic system, plays an important role in brain health and integration.

The star of our superpowers' neurological show appears to be the cingulate cortex, part of the ancient limbic system we learned about in chapter 2. This long area at the very center of our brain lies directly above the corpus callosum and directly below our brain assets.

The cingulate cortex has three major regions that form the cradle of the mind, shown in figure 6.2. The posterior cingulate cortex (PCC), the autobiographical center of the brain, lies toward the back, anchoring the default network and our Story Superpower. The front of the *anterior cingulate cortex* (ACC) works closely with the frontal lobe to generate our Steer Superpower. The back end of the ACC, also called the mid-cingulate, gathers our Self Superpower, working with other key subcortical structures such as the amygdala and insula. As we'll discuss further in chapter 7, the ACC is the part of the brain that is highly developed in Super-Agers, people over 80 who live long and well.

The ACC knits together our health, emotions, social life, and learning. To accomplish this outsized task, the ACC has just the right tool: spindle neurons, the most advanced type of neuron found in our brain, located predominantly in the right hemisphere.

Spindle neurons, also called von Economo neurons, are known as the equivalent of air traffic controllers for our emotions, quickly sharing updates on emotional activity throughout the brain. The only other animals known to have spindle neurons are the great apes, elephants,

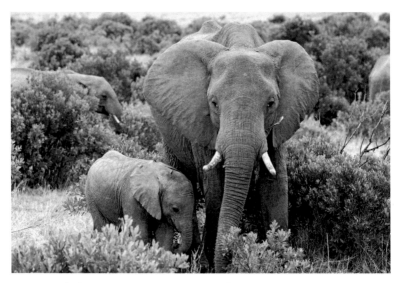

Figure 6.3. Elephants are one of the few species know to have spindle (von Economo) neurons.

and cetaceans. However, humans have more spindle neurons than other species by a very wide margin.

Spindle neurons are also clustered in the insula, which works closely with the ACC to generate our Self Superpower. Working with the invaluable emotional scoop provided by spindle cells, the insula appears to be the command center of behavior, holding a master emotional switch to override the Steer and Story Superpowers as needed to maintain the body's happy place (homeostasis).

Let's consider an example of how our superpowers relate to behavior. At the beginning of the chapter, I mentioned people who have said to me with regard to brain training, "I know what I should do, but I have trouble following through." This inability to follow through suggests the Self Superpower perceives the behavior change to be disadvantageous, and has thrown the master emotional switch to disengage the Steer Superpower. This example could also apply to anyone who has trouble changing behavior for goals such as weight loss or smoking cessation.

When a glitch like this arises, the missing component of our mental activity is *working memory*, the cornerstone of brain health and neuroplasticity.

The crown jewel

Working memory, formerly known as short-term memory, is the crown jewel of our brain's rationally inclined Steer Superpower. This mental scratch pad is part of our brain's learning pipeline, a way station between incoming sensory information in short-term memory and the storage of information in long-term memory. If information doesn't make it into working memory because of exhaustion or emotional interference, the information is not stored in long-term memory, which means that no learning takes place.

But working memory is more than just a vehicle for learning. This cognitive ability allows us to have a fluid mental life and to manipulate new information in conjunction with existing information stored in memory to come up with creative ideas and solutions that are *relevant to the current task that the mind is focused on.*

Some key brain structures related to working memory are the hippocampus, the prefrontal cortex, and the PCC/parietal lobe region. The hippocampus, an important player in all three superpowers, is undermined early in the Alzheimer's disease process. Working memory can easily decline due to inactivity as we get older, leading to cognitive inflexibility, a suspected risk factor for dementia and other age-related psychosocial disorders.

However, working memory can also be toned, like a muscle. People like Captain Chesley Sullenberger prove how valuable working memory can be when it is kept in good shape. On January 15, 2009, US Airways Flight 1549 experienced failure in both engines shortly after takeoff. A skillful response by Captain Sullenberger, then a few days shy of his fifty-eighth birthday, led to a miraculous outcome: he and the crew ditched the plane in the freezing Hudson River with no loss of life.

Reflecting on the initial crash, Captain Sullenberger said, "The physiological reaction I had for this was strong and

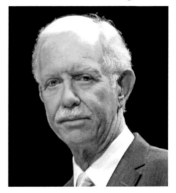

Figure 6.4. Captain Chesley Sullenberger was hailed as a national hero in the United States.

I had to force myself to use my training and force calm on the situation." Once Captain Sullenberger overcame the visceral fear and panic of an imminent crash, his brain was able to sift through stored memories from years of experience for alternatives on the best course of action, given the circumstances. This ability to inhibit emotional responses and the impulsive actions they suggest is the hallmark of a well-trained Steer Superpower.

Working memory enabled Captain Sullenberger to come up with a quick response and instruct the crew to execute the successful rescue plan. His working memory really *worked!* The power of working memory is this ability to transcend time, seamlessly working with information related to the past, present, and future to guide the next step toward a desirable outcome.

Working memory is not useful only in such extreme situations. It is also a helpful companion in daily life, allowing you to remember the names of people you just met, where you parked your car or left your car keys, or the items on the grocery list you wrote out last night and left at home. Memory lapses about these kinds of things are not signs of impending Alzheimer's, but they should not simply be dismissed as normal aging if you want a brain that gets better with age.

My maternal grandmother's working memory was sharp as a tack right before she died from cardiac problems, close to age 90. During my last visit to her home in the woods of central Pennsylvania, I was telling her what good potato salad my boyfriend's mother had made. She asked what was in it. I rattled off a list of nine ingredients, and then left with my mom to run errands for several hours. When we returned, all nine ingredients were on the table, and my grandmother asked me if I would make the potato salad. She had heard me say the ingredients once, and she was nearly blind, yet all the right ingredients were there—and yes, I did make the salad!

This feat made such an impression on me at age 24 that I have never forgotten it, even though I gave no thought to the brain or its abilities way back then. Perhaps because of this formative personal experience, I have always been skeptical about the pronouncements on the inevitabil-

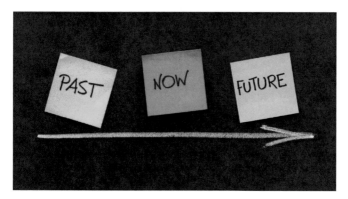

Figure 6.5. Working memory allows our brain to use memory to guide current actions toward a desired future outcome.

ity of age-related cognitive decline and have fought it in myself, kicking and screaming.

Some years ago, I noticed that my working memory, which had been laser-sharp in my early forties, had turned to mush by my late forties. It dawned on me that it could be bad for business to be a brain coach without a strong working memory. So let me share a story about my own trials and triumphs in buffing up my working memory.

The Hands See

In chapter 3, I shared some background about investing in my least active brain asset, the parietal lobe. After five years of fits and starts in attempting to do this, I read an article by a cognitive neuroscientist that said the parietal lobe provided backup storage space to the frontal lobe for working memory. I wondered whether engaging my parietal lobe more actively would improve my working memory. I got excited about trying to meet this challenge—an important sign that my Self Superpower and intrinsic motivation were working for me this time.

My hypothesis was that if I vigorously did something hands-on to engage my parietal lobe, the new synaptic connections would improve my working memory as well. To test my hypothesis, I signed up for a five-day sculpture and drawing class at a local art school, even though I had done no sculpture or drawing since the age of six.

Monday morning I showed up for class. The course description had indicated that the class was for all levels. As it turned out, I was the only beginner in a class of six. There was nowhere to hide. The class began at 9 AM, and by about 10 AM I thought 4 PM could not come soon enough.

The instructor, an internationally acclaimed sculptor, was my exact opposite, a paragon of parietal agility. At first I found him very annoying. I was inept, and he kept reprimanding me, as if he had learned to teach at the school of negative psychology in his native Russia. I resented the criticism. How could he expect me to do something well if I had never done it before? Besides, I was not aiming to make a living as an artist, as he did; I was just after some brain exercise. The first day left me demoralized, wondering if I should quit.

 On the second morning of class, I was trying to sculpt in clay the attractive young nude woman model on a pedestal four feet in front of me. The neck and shoulders were hard to shape. The instructor kept snapping at me with comments like, "That's wrong! Make what you see!"

I kept trying, to no avail. He must have sensed my frustration. He then told me to close my eyes and form the neck and shoulders. In thirty seconds, I was done, and he praised the outcome. I still remember what he said: "The hands see. I don't know how they see, but they see." Since then, I have had this experience many times: the hands "see" in the dark. Unlike the eyes, they are fearless!

By Wednesday morning, two people in the class had already quit, and I was still sorely tempted. But I figured that if I could put up with the instructor's teaching style, I could trust him to deliver what I was after: new skills to form some new synaptic connections in my underactive parietal lobe to improve my working memory.

Fortunately, I spoke some Russian, including some swear words, which made the instructor crack a smile every now and then. Others in the class were very talented, and I also learned from watching them. Eventually, I made drawings and sculptures that weren't half bad for a beginner, as you can see for yourself in figure 6.6. Even he was surprised!

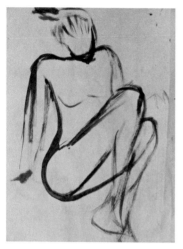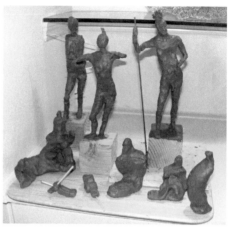

Figure 6.6. The author's drawing and sculptures after a week-long class.

More importantly, I noticed three significant changes in myself during the week. First, even though the class ran for seven hours every day and I spent most of that time standing up, at the end of each day I had so much energy! I figured that since the parietal lobe is in charge of physical sensation, it was revved up by the standing up and hands-on work, filling my brain and body with mojo.

Second, my dreams were wild all that week. I figured that this change was related to the brain's work in building new synaptic connections in my parietal lobe and some unconscious emotional reactions to it.

But the best part was that my working memory was noticeably better by day 4 of this class! On my lunch break that day, I checked my home voice mail, and there was a message from a new appliance-repair person returning my call from two days before, leaving his ten-digit number for a return call. I was in a hurry and had nothing to write with, so I listened to the message once and hung up.

Then I started to dial the guy's number, thinking to myself that if I remembered the number, it would be a miracle. My fingers pushed a series of keys on my cell phone, and next thing I knew, I was talking to the guy who had called! The funny thing was, I didn't "remember" the number; it seemed as though the information floated forward from the back of my mind into my fingers. There was a ghostly feeling about all of this, but I was thrilled. I had grown some new synaptic connections in my parietal lobe, and they were improving my working memory already!

This successful outcome led me to believe that by investing in my least active brain asset, I had converted brain activity in the parietal lobe from *inaccessible* to *accessible* mental activity—and boosted my working memory along the way.

The keys to my success were having a specific goal (improving working memory) and taking a concrete action (going to the class). Before the class, I had tried halfheartedly for five years to work my parietal lobe in other ways, without much payoff. The sculpture instructor, gruff as he was, gave me what I needed to change my ways: a social context for learning.

As we discovered in chapter 2, social context is a major influence on our brain chemistry. When a person feels trust in others, the social bonding neurotransmitter oxytocin flows in the brain and keeps anxiety at bay. Oxytocin is the only neurotransmitter in the brain that is more powerful than dopamine, which drives learning, habits, and addiction.

In the presence of oxytocin, primitive brain areas, including the anterior cingulate cortex, almost magically fire up the superpowers and enable you to go along with the group and learn to do whatever the group is doing.

This well-known phenomenon is known as "unconscious anchoring," "group mind," or "hive mind." The power of group mind can work against us, as is demonstrated by the mass deaths at Jonestown in 1978 or the folktale of the emperor's new clothes. But it can work in our favor, too, as it did for me in the sculpture class.

My approach to improving working memory would not have been so difficult if I had not waited five years to take a class and get the benefits of unconscious anchoring. Even so, it has paid off. People have remarked on my ability to remember names and speak to groups without notes, answering questions without getting off track and still ending on time.

In the years since that sculpture class, I have continued to keep my parietal lobe buffed up. Most recently, I completed a nineteen-mile hike down and up the Grand Canyon over three days, including two nights of

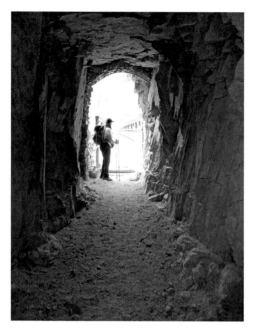

Figure 6.7. During a 19-mile trek in the Grand Canyon, the author gets ready to cross the Black Suspension Bridge over the Colorado River.

camping. This endeavor worked all of my brain assets and engaged my full mental range of motion in the following ways:

Occipital/achievement: the successful completion of the project

Parietal/adventure: camping, encountering the unknown and being in nature 24/7

Temporal/attachment: going with a childhood friend who had suggested the endeavor

Frontal/adaptation: planning ahead and handling unexpected challenges along the way

Default/autobiography: undertaking the greatest test of my physical abilities in my life

After this amazing adventure, my superpowers were all revved up. I could feel it way down deep inside, and my mental clarity reached a new high. My best guess is that being in nature 24/7 and not sitting much gave my whole brain a huge boost. As Henry David Thoreau wrote in *Walking:* "I believe that there is a subtle magnetism in Nature, which, if we unconsciously yield to it, will direct us aright."

Rebalancing the superpowers is hard work, but it is worth it. My working memory is now better at age 57 than it was when I was under 40—and so is my long-term memory, for that matter. My working memory and long-term memory aren't perfect, nor do I expect them to be. When I have a success, I just pat my brain on the head and say, "Way to go," so it knows that was a win and it should do more of that. And it does. I also make it a point to affirm others when their memory works well.

superpowers self-assessment

Now perhaps it is easier to see why our brain is the most complex structure in the world: juggling these superpowers is a big job! To get better with age, we must do what we can to help our brain keep these marvelous powers in balance.

If your superpowers are out of balance, an inner state of unease and emotional turmoil can result, disrupting working memory. Don't worry when this happens. The brain can get in and out of shape like the rest of the body.

However, you need to pay attention to what our brain is telling you. When this imbalance lasts too long, anxiety and isolation may tempt our brain to take the easy way out and prompt us for substances to cope. Here are a few common quick fixes for the chemical imbalance caused by toxic emotions (see the glossary for more information about the role of these neurotransmitters):

> **Alcohol (ethyl):** inhibits glutamate, stimulates release of dopamine and GABA
>
> **Amphetamines:** stimulate dopamine release
>
> **Barbiturates (tranquilizers):** stimulate release of GABA
>
> **Caffeine:** inhibits release of adenosine
>
> **Cannabis (THC, marijuana):** stimulates release of *anandamide,* dopamine, and GABA

Carbohydrates: stimulates release of serotonin

Cocaine: stimulates release of dopamine, norepinephrine, and serotonin

Financial rewards: stimulates release of dopamine (especially unexpected rewards)

LSD: stimulates release of serotonin

MDMA (ecstasy): stimulates release of norepinephrine and serotonin

Nicotine: stimulates release of acetylcholine and dopamine

Opiates (heroin, morphine): stimulate release of dopamine, analgesic endogenous opioids, and GABA

Sugar: stimulates release of serotonin

These substances tend to increase the production of feel-good neurotransmitters, many of which have an analgesic (pain-relieving) or anxiolytic (anxiety-reducing) effect. But since none of these substances enable neuroplasticity (and indeed may inhibit it), they are of little use in getting better with age.

For example, if anxiety keeps you awake at night and you self-medicate with caffeine and nicotine to stay alert during the day, your brain may not have the time or mojo to grow new synaptic connections, a process that takes place mainly during sleep. Or if you are overstimulated in the evening from staring into the screen of a technological device and then use alcohol and carbohydrates to relax, poor sleep and exhaustion can undermine your Steer and Story Superpowers, which use the most resources.

Inadequate sleep is a major derailer of superpower activity and should be avoided at all costs if one wants to get better with age. At night, the *glia*, nannies to the neurons, perform important housekeeping tasks. Originally, glial cells were thought to hold the brain together; the word "glia" comes from the Greek word for "glue." However, glia are now considered the stars of brain health, since they nourish and protect neurons, remove waste, and enable neuroplasticity. Poor-quality nocturnal sleep interferes with these important glial activities. Daytime drowsiness or napping suggests inadequate nighttime sleep.

If you would like to hone your superpowers in ways that support neuroplasticity, begin by using figure 6.8 to assess whether you are using these superpowers to full advantage. As with the brain assets, your best opportunity for personal growth lies in developing your least active superpower. Figure 6.9 provides some activities that can hone the super-powers by building new synaptic connections in the associated brain areas.

While conducting this self-assessment, I would encourage you to for-get about any self-limiting thoughts from the past. The most insidious source of these Steer Superpower derailers is criticism (well-meaning or not) from family, friends, and authority figures leveled against some-one under the age of 12. Since the brain is not fully developed until ages 25–30 and continues to change and grow, any judgments made of you or your capabilities under the age of 12 were premature. For now, just pre-tend these people were wrong about you.

Personality types, gender stereotypes (men can't do this, women can't do that), and racial stereotypes are also not helpful for this exer-cise. There is no basis for such self-limiting beliefs in scientific research or real life. The focus should be on what we *are* capable of, and every human being is capable of accessing these three superpowers—even if half of the brain is removed, as we learned from Albert and Robert in chapter 3. You are the captain of your own soul in building out the blue-print of your life.

If you aren't sure which superpower to work on, I suggest you start with the Self Superpower. Remember, the Steer Superpower is a coordi-nator of brain resources to achieve desirable outcomes; it does not orig-inate desires and motives but develops a plan for following through on them. Without input from the Self and Story Superpowers, the Steer Superpower is spinning its wheels.

The most frequent advice that I give to others consists of six words: "Take a class" and "Try something new." Learn from my mistakes. Take an in-person class and not an online class if at all possible, to get the ben-efits of oxytocin in building new synaptic connections. Contact a local library, adult school, community college, or retreat center in your area for information about classes. If you don't know what some of the suggestions in figure 6.9 are, ask a friend, a holistic practitioner, or a cleric.

As a general rule of thumb, stay away from screens (movie, television, computer, tablet, phone, etc.) when trying to sharpen your superpowers. Also, reading is of little value in this regard, unless it is in preparation for a group discussion. Technology and reading are like a sensory deprivation chamber for our brain, which is particularly taxing for our Self Superpower.

But why bother to train the brain for an hour and then work against it the rest of the day? Ultimately, our lifestyle must encourage neuroplasticity if we are to keep our superpowers in balance to live long and well. So now we will meet the most successful people in the world, cognitively speaking, to learn their secrets for maintaining neuroplasticity well beyond age 80.

Beware of illness as much as you can, so that as far as possible your self
is not the cause of any weakness . . . So for the love of God
control your body and soul alike with great care,
and keep as fit as you can.
The Cloud of Unknowing, author unknown

Figure 6.8. superpowers self-assessment

1. Under each superpower, assess your current strength in each activity listed using a scale of 1 to 10, with 1 being low and 10 being high.

2. Use the same scale to indicate an overall score for each superpower in the blanks below.

SELF: _____

STORY: _____

STEER: _____

I. SELF SUPERPOWER: SENSORY-MOTOR SKILLS
Focus: Integrating personal experiences and relationships
Assess your current strength of each ability/activity listed using a scale of 1 to 10, with 1 being low and 10 being high.

_____ 1. Having sensory experiences that induce awe or an appreciation of beauty or harmony

_____ 2. Maintaining daily routines that promote good health with regard to nutrition, exercise, relaxation, hygiene, sleep, learning, creativity, encounters with nature, social activity, financial order, work, and service to others

_____ 3. Accepting personal emotional and/or physical pain, and finding ways to manage or eliminate it

_____ 4. Cultivating friendships outside of work that include affection, conversation, fun, humor, reciprocity, smiling, and trust

_____ 5. Exercising self-expression (non-verbal), such as art or cooking

_____ 6. Being in touch with the desires of the heart and yearnings for unfulfilled hopes and dreams

II. STORY SUPERPOWER: THEORY OF MIND SKILLS

Focus: Understanding the mental states of self and others

Assess your current strength in each activity listed using a scale of 1 to 10, with 1 being low and 10 being high.

_____ 1. Recognizing intentional movements in other people
Identifying other people as agents of intentional actions
Recognizing their goals
Assessing their intentions

_____ 2. Sharing the intentional movements of others
Imitation
Mimicry
Automatic empathy

_____ 3. Sharing the intentional mental activity of others
Joint attention: looking at something together
Visual perspective taking: seeing how another sees
Understanding the desires and goals that motivate others

_____ 4. Inferring the mental state of others, including current emotional activity and feelings

_____ 5. Anticipating how others might act, given their mental states

_____ 6. Simulating alternative scenarios: figuring out what someone might have done differently to get a better outcome

_____ 7. Using information about mental states to predict outcomes and to simulate alternative scenarios for one's own behavior

_____ 8. Identifying incongruities between intentions and outcomes that convey humor

_____ 9. Verbal self-scripting: developing narratives to explain behavior of self, others, and the world at large

III. STEER SUPERPOWER: EXECUTIVE FUNCTION SKILLS

Focus: Voluntary, nonroutinized thinking and behavior

Assess your current strength of each ability/activity listed using a scale of 1 to 10, with 1 being low and 10 being high.

_____ 1. Self-regulation: directing the use of cognitive capacities (including reasoning, language, visual and spatial information, and memory) to achieve desirable outcomes

* Attention—maintaining sustained concentration on tasks

* Behavioral change—modifying actions to achieve a goal

* Choice—using subjective values to express a preference

* Emotion regulation—control and management of emotions

* Flexibility—adapting to circumstances, including problem solving

* Inhibitory control—stopping a behavior or resisting an impulse

* Initiation—beginning tasks or projects without being prompted

* Learning—adding new information to memory

* Organization—managing personal effects and work

* Planning—developing strategies to accomplish tasks

* Self-monitoring—self-evaluation and correction of behavior

* Self-talk—internalizing self-directed speech for behavior within constraints or rules

* Working memory—retaining and manipulating distinct pieces of information over short periods of time, while resisting interfering information and managing emotional responses

_____ 2. Self-realization: understanding personal strengths and challenges and how one's own behavior affects others

_____ 3. Self-determination: developing a personal set of meaningful goals and long-term plans that motivate and drive behavior

_____ 4. Self-awareness: understanding personal motives (why do I do the things I do?)

_____ 5. Self-transcendence: contemplating life's meaning (where am I from? why am I here? what is the meaning of life?)

Figure 6.9. Activities for Honing the Superpowers

I. SELF SUPERPOWER:
promote safety, trust, and a mind-body connection

Art (drawing, painting, sculpting)
Caring for animals or babies
Cooking for supportive family and friends
Dancing
Deep breathing
Drumming
Equine therapy
Games of chance in a group (backgammon, bingo, board games)
Gardening
Gratitude attitude
Holistic therapies (aromatherapy, reflexology, etc.)
Mandala drawing
Massage
Playfulness
Prayer (from the heart)
Talking to a trusted friend
Walking a labyrinth
Yoga

II. STORY SUPERPOWER:
promote psychosocial engagement and verbal access to mental states

Acting
Attending a live performance (theater, dance, music)
Games involving teamwork (charades, Jenga)
Identifying unfulfilled yearnings
Improvisation in a group
Learning a new language in a class
Listening to music from your teens and 20s
Preaching
Singing
Small group discussion of personal or spiritual matters

Small group fiction book study and discussion
Stand-up comedy
Play reading in a group
Playing a musical instrument
Writing your own obituary
Writing workshop (autobiographical or creative writing)

III. STEER SUPERPOWER:
promote self-awareness and emotional regulation

"Can't" therapy (do something you think you can't do)
Confession of guilt
Debate club
Discussion group for current events or nonfiction books
Dream workshop
Examen of consciousness practice
Games of strategy (bridge, chess)
Gratitude journal
Launching a new group or project for the common good
Meditation or centering prayer (individual or group)
Mindfulness training
Personal retreat
Public speaking
Setting personal goals and a plan to achieve them
Tai chi

Engagement Questions

1. Which of the three superpowers is your strong suit: Self, Story, or Steer? Who are the positive and negative role models for you in building this strength?

2. Which of the three superpowers do you struggle with the most: Self, Story, or Steer? Who are the positive and negative role models for you in this struggle?

3. Are any of the substances on the self-medication list a challenge for you? Why is this, and who can help you successfully meet this challenge?

4. What attitudes about money did you grow up with (for example, "money doesn't grow on trees" or "you can't take it with you")? How do these attitudes help or hinder your relationship with money today?

5. If your superpowers need rebalancing at this time, which activity from figure 6.9 might work best for you?

6. How would you answer these questions to frame your personal narrative:

   Whom have I loved, and who has loved me?

   Whom have I served, and who has served me?

   What have I accomplished in my life that I am proud of?

   What losses have left me with open emotional wounds that need to heal?

   Is my life a series of gains and losses that are trending up or trending down?

   How have I shared my wisdom with the next generation?

   If I died today, what would my legacy be? Would there be any regrets or unfinished business from my life?

CHAPTER 7

The Better with Age Lifestyle

 The goal of life is to make your heartbeat match the beat of the universe, to match your nature with Nature. JOSEPH CAMPBELL

I n this chapter, we will consider the elements of a lifestyle that will help us get better with age. This type of lifestyle, which promotes neuroplasticity as a matter of routine, gives us the best shot at living both long *and* well, as Picasso did.

For some two hundred thousand years, some members of our species have succeeded at living long and well. Wouldn't it be great if by now we had some solid scientific evidence of how to keep our brains healthy, applicable to people of all ages and from all cultures? Unfortunately, such evidence does not yet exist.

However, since the beginning of the twentieth century, some fifty Nobel prizes have been awarded for breakthroughs in neuroscience. These advances have brought us some important findings about our brain.

As we discovered at the beginning of this learning adventure, the good news for everyone is that a healthy brain is designed to improve with age, like a bottle of fine wine. Until recently, the scientific view was that neuroplasticity ended well before gray hair appeared. Over the past few years, evidence from several major studies, brain-imaging technology, and real-life outcomes have confirmed that neuroplasticity continues throughout the human life span. This evidence has triggered a huge paradigm shift among neuroscientists about how the brain ages.

And now the bad news. This three-pound wonder brain of ours is not only the most complex structure in the known universe but the most mysterious as well. As a result, when something goes wrong, effective interventions can be elusive.

Despite all the accomplishments of neuroscience, huge gaps remain in understanding how the brain works. Important questions remain unanswered: What keeps the brain healthy? What derails neuroplasticity? Impaired neuroplasticity is associated with numerous neurological disorders, particularly dementia.

A Brain check-up

One of the most troubling brain malfunctions of our times is Alzheimer's disease, the most common form of dementia. Dementia is a condition that has long been associated with age, hence the term *senile dementia*. In 1906, Dr. Alois Alzheimer of Frankfurt, Germany, first reported the condition of *presenile dementia*, a disease he had observed for five years in a German woman until her death at age 56. When he performed an autopsy, he observed abnormalities in her brain tissue: clumps and fragments known as amyloid plaques and neurofibrillary tangles.

Some one hundred years later, it is still not clear whether these plaques and tangles are a cause or an effect of the disease. For example, the Alzheimer's researcher David Snowdon discusses the results of a study he conducted among U.S. nuns in his book *Aging with Grace: What the Nun Study Teaches Us about Leading Longer, Healthier, and More Meaningful Lives.* The book, published in 2002, revealed that some nuns with excellent cognitive function in their 90s had abundant plaques and tangles in their brains that were discovered by autopsy. Apparently, neuroplasticity allows the brain to work around the dead neurons associated with plaques and tangles.

Research has also failed to find a smoking genetic gun for Alzheimer's. Fewer than 5 percent of Alzheimer's cases can be explained by inherited genes. In these individuals, symptoms typically begin well before age 50, with death often occurring before age 60, as with Dr. Alzheimer's original patient. In the other 95 percent of Alzheimer's cases, the disease is triggered by *epigenetic* factors—disturbances of genetic activity triggered by factors related to behavior, culture, environment, lifestyle, and stress. But the specific triggers of the disease have eluded researchers.

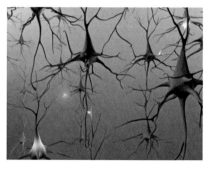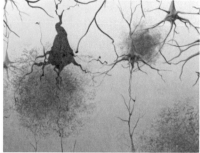

Figure 7.1. Alzheimer's cells (shown on the right) are surrounded by plaque deposits that disrupt communication with other cells. Healthy cells (shown on the left) do not have these deposits.

The only known risk factor for Alzheimer's is age: a ten-year-old can get cancer, but not Alzheimer's. This may in part be due to the delayed development of the target of Alzheimer's—the default network brain asset, seat of our Story Superpower—which does not mature until after age 40.

The other possible contributing factors you may have heard about— diet, educational level, exercise, gender—are scientific guesses, backed only by wobbly correlations rather than direct causal evidence. A significant contributing factor to Alzheimer's that you may not have heard of is culture. Alzheimer's rates vary greatly by state in the United States, and by country around the world.

Understandably, many people over fifty are alarmed about the prospect of dementia. In 2010, I attended a lecture by a Columbia University Alzheimer's researcher titled "Alzheimer's and the Aging Brain." During the Q&A session, a woman asked a good question: "We go to the doctor to get a check-up for our heart, blood, bones, and other things. Can't we get a brain check-up too?" The researcher said no, not yet. There still isn't one.

Perhaps we will have the equivalent of a brain check-up some day. Efforts such as the BRAIN Initiative, the Human Connectome Project, and the European Commission's Human Brain Project may generate a whole new understanding of the brain many years from now. However, at this point, no one knows why some people get Alzheimer's and others don't. The disease is still difficult to diagnose, and effective medical treatments remain elusive.

Neuroscientists widely agree on one piece of commonsense advice for a healthy brain: use it or lose it. But the research trail runs cold on the best ways to "use it." Exercises such as computer-based brain training games have been renounced by many neuroscientists as an ineffective tool for improving cognitive health.

Until medical research can deliver more certain answers, we can learn something from a special class of people who are aging like Picasso: the Super-Agers, who manage to *live long and well.* These seniors follow a lifestyle that has helped them retain neuroplasticity and get better with age. They are not losing it, so let's consider how they are using it.

If we knew what it was we were doing, it would not be called research, would it?

ALBERT EINSTEIN

The Brain secrets of super-Agers

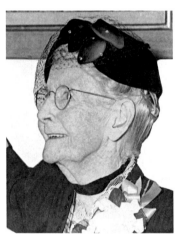

Figure 7.2. Grandma Moses in 1952, at age 92.

A famous twentieth-century Super-Ager is Grandma Moses. Anna Mary Robertson Moses, nicknamed Grandma Moses, was a renowned American folk artist. She was born on a farm in New York in 1860, the year before the Civil War began. Widowed after a full life of farming and raising children, she had to give up embroidery and quilting at age 76 due to arthritis. At her sister Celestia's suggestion, she tried painting. She loved the way art allowed her to make something out of nothing without needing raw materials.

Grandma Moses' art was discovered by a collector in 1938, and within a few years she became a worldwide sensation. She painted over 1,500 canvases in twenty-five years and died with her boots on at the age of

101. Her physician said the cause of her death was that she just wore out. A U.S. postal stamp honoring Grandma Moses was issued posthumously in 1969.

But not all Super-Agers are famous. Over the years, I have met many people who have lived long and well—perhaps you have, too. I have already mentioned examples from my family: my maternal grandmother and father-in-law. Another noteworthy example is a couple I met almost 20 years ago.

One sunny afternoon, as my husband Peter and I were moving into our new home in Arizona, our next-door neighbors stopped by to introduce themselves and drop off a warm casserole for dinner. Henry, a retired corporate lawyer, and his wife, Shirley, were both Midwesterners in their eighties.

We all enjoyed getting to know one another over the next few months. Two years later, Henry and Shirley sold their home and moved into the independent living section of a nearby continuing-care retirement community. We figured this was something like a nursing home, and they were going there to die. However, the opposite happened: after the move, they began to live even better, becoming more alert and lively. Some fifteen years later, Henry and Shirley are still at that retirement community, living independently and pushing one hundred years old.

I never thought of Henry and Shirley as cognitively special until I learned about the SuperAging research study being conducted at the Cognitive Neurology and Alzheimer's Disease Center at Northwestern University.

Initiated in 2010, the study aims to discover what is going right with Super-Agers, the people like Henry and Shirley who remain active, adventurous, creative, energetic, independent, resilient, sociable, and wise well past age 80. The researchers hope to identify their aging secrets and to determine whether these factors can be learned and emulated by others.

As of August 2013, the research team had recruited four hundred volunteers age 80 or over who were mentally sharp and living independently. They screened the volunteers using several parameters, including cognitive function; only 35 of the 400 volunteers met their standards for participating in the study.

The study is still ongoing, but the research team has already made an important discovery from the elite seniors who made the grade. Referred to as Super-Agers, these people had fewer age-related plaques than those who did not qualify for the study.

In addition, the thirty-five Super-Agers who qualified for the study had more mass in the anterior cingulate cortex (ACC) than most people in their fifties and sixties! These preliminary findings suggest that the primitive, socially oriented ACC, discussed in chapter 6, is the integrating force of a brain that gets better with age.

The ACC is the anchor of our Self and Steer superpowers. Equipped with powerful spindle neurons, the ACC works with the frontal lobe to knit together our emotions, health, social lives, and experiences of pain (emotional, social, and physical). The ACC's duties include these key cognitive functions:

Appraisal of emotional stimulus
Attention
Conflict resolution
Decision making
Emotional expression
Emotional regulation
Empathy
Error detection
Impulse control
Pain perception
Regulation of autonomic body functions
Reward anticipation

By maintaining neuroplasticity in the pivotal ACC region, these Super-Agers' brains were getting better with age. Perhaps the Super-Agers' secret lies deep within the connections of the ACC: the use of rationality and pleasurable interpersonal interaction to protect brain cells from toxic emotions, pain (be it emotional or physical in origin), and inflammation.

Surprisingly, the Super-Agers do not necessarily follow all the healthy lifestyle rules that are touted as Alzheimer's prevention measures. Those in the study didn't all eat healthy foods; some of them smoked and drank. They didn't all graduate from college. Nevertheless, they all stayed engaged with people and life: they were happy to be alive. They focused on gain, not loss.

If the Super-Agers are not losing it, presumably they must be using it in the ways that count. But they're not doing special brain-training activity. Neuroplasticity is built into their lifestyle, which is the ultimate form of brain training.

However, lifestyle choices do not arise in a vacuum. Some communities make it easier to live a brain-friendly lifestyle than others. When it comes to diet, you are what you eat. When it comes to neuroplasticity, you are where you live. Just as a bottle of fine wine is infused with the *terroir*—the soil, climate, and wine-making techniques—of where the grapes are grown, so our brains are steeped in the nature and culture of where we live.

where the super-agers are

People in different places have different philosophies and ways of living. Daily lifestyles vary tremendously from one country to another, as I learned firsthand from studying abroad during college.

In 1977, I spent the summer at the University of Urbino in Italy, taking classes in Italian language and culture to earn eight college credits. Urbino is a medieval hilltop town in the Apennine Mountains well east of Florence, a short bus ride from the Adriatic coast. The slow pace of life in this hilltop town was a disappointment to our group of college students. The town was proud of its most famous native son, the Renaissance artist Raphael. However, we were quick to observe that Raphael had had the sense to leave at the age of fourteen and never come back.

Even so, that summer in Urbino was memorable. Church bells marked the rhythm of the day for everyone. Walking was the only way to

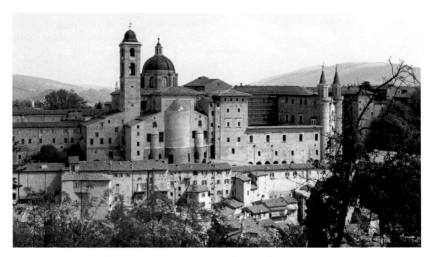

Figure 7.3. Urbino, Italy, is a medieval city on a hilltop in the Apennine Mountains.

get around the narrow, winding stone streets of the inner city, where we lived and attended school. In the early afternoon, the smells of home-cooked meals and the sounds of silverware clinking against plates wafted through the open windows as we walked by.

Everyone was very friendly to us. On our way home from class in the heat of the day, we would often stop at a little mom-and-pop gelato shop on a steep hill near our school and practice our Italian. The owners insisted we try gelato made from fresh local figs.

Buying something from a store was a major challenge. The first hurdle was getting inside: the stores were open in the morning while I was in school, closed between noon and 4 P.M. when I was out of school, and then open again when we were busy with dinner and evening activities. Few of the storekeepers spoke English, so my fledgling Italian and sign language had to do.

The whole town had only one television, located in a public building. I still remember walking by that glass-walled room, filled with fifteen or twenty people watching a talk show on a small black-and-white TV hanging from the ceiling. I wondered how they could decide on what to watch without fighting.

By late afternoon, all the action was in the town's central piazza. Every day, people of all ages gathered in that square, talking, laughing.

smoking, drinking, eating, flirting, and listening to music, with kids running around playing, as if it were a giant outdoor living room. What's the point? I wondered. Don't they find it boring to hang out in the same place with the same people every day? Life in Italy seemed to revolve around family, friends, food, fun, conversation, art, and music. In my New Jersey hometown, study, sports, reading, movies, shopping, and a part-time job played a bigger role in my daily life as a teenager.

Back then, I wasn't thinking about neuroplasticity. But decades later, when I learned that Italians live a few years longer on average than Americans and have an Alzheimer's rate some 60 percent lower, I thought back to the marked cultural differences I had noticed there as a teenager. Italy is better at producing Super-Agers than many other countries, including the United States.

Let's take a closer look at which cultures grow the most bountiful harvests of Super-Agers. First we will consider longevity. Mirror, mirror, on the wall, who lives the longest of them all? The international study *U.S. Health in International Perspective: Shorter Lives, Poorer Health,* released in 2013 by the National Research Council and Institute of Medicine of the National Academies, compared health and life expectancy outcomes for seventeen high-income countries for the period 2004-7.

Not surprisingly, this study found that people in high-income countries live longer, on average, than people elsewhere. Also, women tend to live longer than men, by three to seven years, in the 17 high-income countries in the study.

As figure 7.4 indicates, the people who live the longest in the study—and in the world—are Japanese women, with a life expectancy at birth of almost eighty-six years. They outlive Japanese men by about seven years and American men by ten years. Switzerland's men live the longest at 79.33 years, followed closely by Australian men (79.27 years) and Japanese men (79.20 years).

In addition to Japan, other countries that rank highly for both male and female longevity include Australia, Italy, and Switzerland.

Surprisingly, the United States is at the bottom of this high-income heap when it comes to longevity. According to the study, Americans lag not just in the length of their life spans, but also in quality of life.

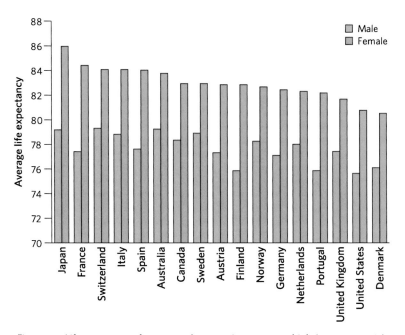

Figure 7.4. Life expectancy for men and women in seventeen high-income countries.

Americans who make it to age 50 arrive there with more debilitating and costly health impairments than the residents of other high-income countries.

Poorer health outcomes in the United States do not result from lower spending on health care. Americans spend twice as much on health care as any of the other countries studied. The study cites "inefficiencies in the U.S. healthcare system" as a major factor in the last-place showing of the United States.

However, flaws in the health-care system do not tell the whole story. According to the study, the disappointing state of Americans' health has complex origins:

No single factor can fully explain the U.S. health disadvantage. Deficiencies in the health care system may worsen illnesses and increase deaths from certain diseases, but they cannot explain the nation's higher rates of traffic accidents or violence. Similarly, although individual behaviors are clearly important, they do not

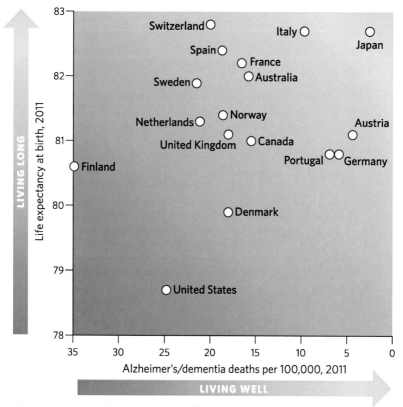

Figure 7.5. Average life expectancy and Alzheimer's/dementia death rates in seventeen high-income countries.

explain why Americans who do not smoke or are not overweight also appear to have higher rates of disease than similar groups in peer countries. More likely, the U.S. health disadvantage has multiple causes and involves some combination of inadequate health care, unhealthy behaviors, adverse economic and social conditions, and environmental factors, as well as public policies and social values that shape those conditions.

Now let's consider the "living well" aspect of super-aging. For simplicity, our measure of living well will be the rate of Alzheimer's or dementia deaths per 100,000 of population on an age-standardized basis. Figure 7.5 shows both the average life expectancy and the Alzheimer's/dementia

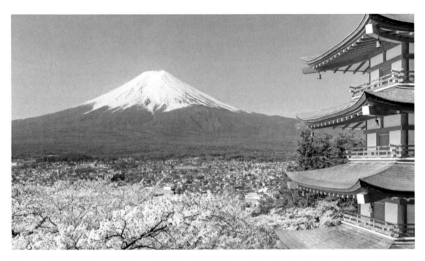

Figure 7.6. Mt. Fuji, one of Japan's "Three Holy Mountains," is located 60 miles southwest of Tokyo.

death rate for the same seventeen high-income countries in the *U.S. Health in International Perspective* study.

Since the Japanese live longer and have one of the oldest societies in the world (median age of 46.1), it would be reasonable to expect that Japan would have a higher rate of Alzheimer's than other countries. Yet Japan has the lowest rate of Alzheimer's deaths compared to other high-income countries by a wide margin. Other countries that have low rates of Alzheimer's deaths include Austria, Germany, Italy, and Portugal.

Given this information, Japan and Italy could be said to have the best cultural soil in the world for growing Super-Agers. This is not to say that Japan and Italy are better than any other countries, and have no problems—far from it. Nor should they rest on their laurels; in 30 years, Japan and Italy might be on the bottom of the high-income country heap, rather than the top. However, they deserve credit for building post–World War II secular societies that promote health and neuroplasticity, especially considering they lost the war.

The United States accounts for only 5 percent of the world's population but has a whopping 20 percent of global Alzheimer's deaths, about ten times the Japanese rate, even though the United States has a younger population with a median age close to 37. Only Finland and Iceland have higher rates of Alzheimer's than the United States, followed closely by Sweden (ranked fourth) and Switzerland (ranked sixth).

Within the United States, there are significant regional disparities in life expectancy and Alzheimer's rates as well. On an age-adjusted basis, the residents of Hawaii, New York, and New Jersey enjoy better odds of living long and well than the residents in the states of Washington, Oregon, or California.

What cultural factors could account for such pronounced differences in longevity and Alzheimer's rates around the world and within the United States? In my experience, Americans are quick to think of diet. They attribute low Alzheimer's rates to something you can put into your mouth: the green tea and sushi in Japan, or the red wine and Mediterranean diet in Italy.

Including fruits, vegetables, and healthy fats in the diet is important. However, echoing the preliminary findings of Northwestern's Super-Aging Study, several landmark studies suggest that something else accounts for super-aging success: not what goes into your mouth, but what goes into your mind.

The Diet of the Mind

In the SuperAging study we considered earlier in this chapter, researchers found that differences between Super-Agers and their peers were not limited to the brain. Super-Agers have more vitality than most people their age, maintaining romantic relationships and a positive, inquisitive outlook on life.

This is not because Super-Agers have better luck or better genes than the rest of us. At least one of the Super-Agers in the study was a concentration camp survivor. They have had their share of losses, big and small.

But what Super-Agers do have is *resilience*, the ability to bounce back from difficulties, moving from loss to gain with a combination of inner strength and social support. Super-Agers don't allow loss to define them as losers. They appear to spend less time on *rumination*, the constant chewing on a negative emotional cud that is associated with anxiety, depression, and chronic inflammation.

So how can we build resilience? According to the website of the American Psychological Association, resilience comes not primarily from diet, exercise, or good genes but from "having caring and supportive relationships within and outside the family. Relationships that create love and trust, provide role models and offer encouragement and reassurance help bolster a person's resilience."

But caring and supportive social relationships are not always available when you need them. What other sources of resilience exist?

William James, the Harvard professor known as the father of American psychology and a mentor to Sigmund Freud and Carl Jung, believed that our relationship with a higher power mattered more than anything else, and that the absence of faith brings physical distress and death. According to James, faith in *something*, and a feeling of being connected to something greater than ourselves, plays an important *biological* function. James cited the potent combination of faith-states and creeds as one of the most important biological functions of mankind.

David Snowdon's nun study, mentioned earlier in this chapter, revealed a strong link between aging well and emotional expression. The study examined autobiographical essays from most of the nuns, dating as far back as their twenties, and concluded that positive emotions expressed in the essays, along with their ability to write about ideas and not only facts, were associated with living long and well. According to our Brain Portfolio Tool, these abilities are linked to the temporal lobe asset (attachment) and the default network asset (autobiography).

We've come full circle, back to the "It's the relationships, stupid" theme from *The Richest of Fare* that I first shared with you at the beginning of our journey. Perhaps when all is said and done, and all the research has been completed, we are never going to find better advice for brain health and resilience than the Golden Rule from Luke 6:31: "Do to others as you would have them do to you."

The only thing that counts is faith
expressing itself through love.
GALATIANS 5:6

Reclaiming Our Brain's Generativity

So what can we do here in the United States to boost neuroplasticity and get better with age? For starters, we need to consider whether our modern lifestyle has pulled the rug out from under our brain.

In chapter 2, we learned about how our brain changes throughout life to support activities in the three main stages of our lives. In traditional societies, people had the basic cognitive skills they needed at puberty to raise children and make an economic contribution to the group. They became grandparents in their mid to late twenties and helped young parents with raising children, right when the frontal lobe was reaching full development. People became great-grandparents in their late thirties and early forties, as the default network became more active, diverting resources from physical activity to brain activity to enable wisdom for the common good.

The most advanced and least efficient brain regions—the frontal lobe and default network—developed at later ages to ensure the survival of the species. Only the few people who lived past age 40 diverted cognitive resources from reproduction and economic activities to integration. These individuals could share their wisdom for the benefit of the whole community, not just their immediate family members.

The multigenerational living arrangements of our hunter-gatherer and agrarian ancestors capitalized on all of our brain's strengths at different ages to aid group survival. By making use of cognitive strengths at different ages, our resource-guzzling brain was able to pull its weight and justify its existence. This pattern of neurological development must have been highly adaptive for some two hundred thousand years.

However, since World War II, the United States has largely abandoned the extended family model, replacing it with some new patterns of living:

Exposure to environmental chemicals and medications that
  disrupt gastrointestinal health
Inadequate high-quality sleep
Less time spent with friends and service organizations
Living far away from family

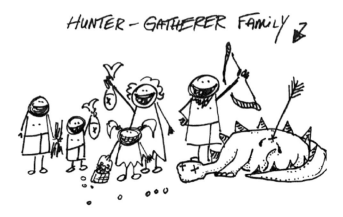

HUNTER - GATHERER FAMILY

Living in over-55 retirement communities
Parents raising young children without the aid of grandparents
and elders
Preference for animals over humans as household members
Reduced interpersonal interaction at home and work due to
electronic devices
Sedentary living
Self-medication with food and drugs to mask toxic emotions
Single-person households

Fortunately, our species excels at adaptation: we don't have to live the way our ancestors lived. However, we have to respect reality. These sea changes in social structure and lifestyle have occurred faster than our brain can adapt.

The American Dream has built the largest economy in the world, leaving a neurological nightmare in its wake. American cultural values emphasize achievement (particularly financial success) and adventure at the expense of relationships and meaning and purpose in life. Not coincidentally, the marginalized brain assets associated with attachment and autobiography are the first areas attacked by Alzheimer's disease.

To boost neuroplasticity, we must use our full mental range of motion. Building language skills at all ages needs to move up on our list of cultural priorities. We need to care for our brain as a valuable asset—more valuable than money—and stop wasting it on fast food and foot-

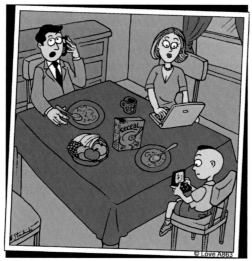
Technology continues to improve communication.

ball, meanness and medications, pollution and pornography, violence and vulgarity.

If I were a betting person, I'd place my bet on the United States stepping up to meet this formidable brain wealth challenge by embracing a new and improved American Dream: life, liberty, and the pursuit of neuroplasticity. As Winston Churchill supposedly once said, "You can always count on the Americans to do the right thing—after they have tried everything else."

Returning to Port

In our learning adventure, we have covered a lot of ground. We learned about neuroplasticity and our brain's back story. We discovered ways to use our brain assets so we don't lose them. We have received tips from many people who have succeeded at building their brain wealth, including the amazing Super-Agers. And we have learned about the overriding importance of social engagement and culture for neuroplasticity at all ages.

As our physical powers wane, our superpowers must compensate to help us get better with age. When the body, mind, spirit, and soul pull together to promote health, our brains are well equipped to stave off the biggest enemy of neuroplasticity: toxic stress and emotions that can lead to chronic inflammation.

The ultimate form of brain training is living a generative lifestyle centered on the deepest roots of our being—one that helps us answer the 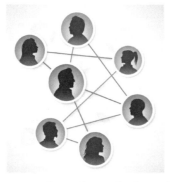 questions: who am I? why am I here? whom do I love? who loves me? how can I help make the universe a friendly place for someone else?

A generative life over age 40 produces a win-win situation for the individual and society: a triumphant autobiography crowned by wisdom, shared to benefit the common good. From this position of strength, we have the best chances of aging like Picasso and the Super-Agers so we can live long and prosper.

You now have a whole new toolkit to manage your brain assets like a well-balanced portfolio, built on the foundation of these seven interwoven threads:

* Full range of mental motion
* Happy gut bacteria
* Healthy, long telomeres
* Integration of inner and outer lives
* Meaning and purpose in serving others
* Neuroplasticity
* Warm, intimate relationships

I hope you have found what you were looking for in *Better with Age,* and that you are more excited than ever about our brain. Now it is time for you to get your superpowers in gear and *do something* with what you have learned so your brain and your life can keep getting better with age.

Farewell, my adventurous friend! Thank you for trusting me to be your guide throughout these pages. May your ship have a following wind as you go forward fearlessly to continue narrating your triumphant life story.

To know and love one other human being
is the root of all wisdom.
EVELYN WAUGH, *Brideshead Revisited*

engagement questions

1. From your experience, what do you think are the most important lifestyle factors that enable people to live long and well? What factors do you think contribute most to developing Alzheimer's disease?

2. Do you know any Super-Agers? What do you admire about them?

3. Have you been to any of the seventeen high-income countries mentioned in this chapter? What differences have you noticed between different countries?

4. Why do you think the United States ranks so low relative to other high-income countries with regard to life expectancy and Alzheimer's/dementia?

5. If you are from outside the United States, what lifestyle differences do you see between your native country and the United States, and how might these differences affect health outcomes?

6. Have you navigated the midlife transition? What wisdom would you share from this experience?

7. What steps do you take to defuse toxic emotions and avoid rumination?

8. What are the three most important insights you have gained from *Better with Age?* How will you act on them?

THEY shall arise in the States,

They shall report Nature, laws, physiology, and happiness;

They shall illustrate Democracy and the kosmos;

They shall be alimentive, amative, perceptive;

They shall be complete women and men—their pose brawny and supple, their drink water, their blood clean and clear;

They shall enjoy materialism and the sight of products—they shall enjoy the sight of the beef, lumber, bread-stuffs, of Chicago, the great city;

They shall train themselves to go in public to become orators and oratresses;

Strong and sweet shall their tongues be—poems and materials of poems shall come from their lives—they shall be makers and finders;

Of them, and of their works, shall emerge divine conveyers, to convey gospels;

Characters, events, retrospections, shall be convey'd in gospels —Trees, animals, waters, shall be convey'd,

Death, the future, the invisible faith, shall all be convey'd.

WALT WHITMAN, FROM *Leaves of Grass*

A Look Ahead

And now these three remain: faith, hope and love.
But the greatest of these is love. I CORINTHIANS 13:13

Before we part, let's consider an unanswered question: Why did Mother Nature work so hard to come up with a brain like ours?

I would so enjoy exploring this question with you, but our time runs short. Our brain assets are awaiting some active management! As Albert Einstein warned, "Anyone who reads too much and uses his own brain too little falls into lazy habits of thinking."

To cut to the chase, let's just pretend Mother Nature did begin with the end in mind when she began developing our brain, and that it is a work in progress. What are her expectations for how we should use our brain assets, mental range of motion, and superpowers? Where are we headed in our evolutionary journey as a species?

I encourage you to use our brain and figure it out for yourself. In the meantime, on the opposite page is the best answer I have come across, from Walt Whitman's *Leaves of Grass,* envisioning a new breed of people.

To these lines I would add:

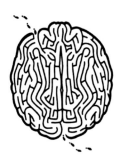

They shall be complete women and men.
They shall make the universe a friendly place.
They shall be called Homo sapiens sapiens amatus.

acetylcholine: A compound made from acetic acid and choline. A major neurotransmitter and the first to be discovered (in 1914), it facilitates muscle movement and vagus nerve/parasympathetic nervous system functions. In the central nervous system, it plays a key role in arousal, sustained attention, learning, memory, neuroplasticity, perception of reward, and rapid eye movement (REM) sleep.

amygdala: Part of the limbic system, an almond-shaped pair of structures located toward the front of the inner temporal lobes. It performs a principal role in the processing of autonomic functions, memory, decision making, emotional reactions, rewards, and sexual behavior.

anandamide: A feel-good neurotransmitter derived from arachidonic acid that occurs naturally in the human brain and in some foods (including chocolate). Anandamide, from the Sanskrit word for "bliss," binds to the same brain receptors as the cannabinoids.

anterior cingulate cortex: A large structure at the center of the brain directly under the upper layer of the cortex. It is part of both the limbic system and the cerebral cortex, integrating the activity of lower, more primitive brain structures with the most advanced activity of the cerebral cortex.

attachment: Strong feelings of affection or loyalty for someone or something.

autonomic nervous system: A major branch of the *peripheral nervous system*, lying outside of the skull and spine and managing homeostasis. Its two major components are the sympathetic nervous system (which mobilizes energy resources to deal with threats) and the parasympathetic nervous system (which conserves energy resources at quiet times). It acts as a control system to direct bodily functions such as breathing, heart rate, blood pressure, digestion, peristalsis, pupillary response, urination, reflex actions (including coughing, sneezing, swallowing, and vomiting), and sexual arousal and orgasm. It is associated with the fight-or-flight response.

axon: The long, thin, tubular structure that carries information away from the cell body of a neuron toward the synapse for transmission to other neurons.

basal ganglia: A collection of structures situated deep within the brain that organize motor behavior and select the appropriate action. The basal ganglia are strongly interconnected with the prefrontal cortex, thalamus, brain stem, cerebellum, and other key brain areas. They are also associated with emotions, procedural learning, routine behaviors, and involuntary habits such as teeth grinding during sleep.

brain stem: A structure that forms the central core of the brain and connects the brain to the spinal cord and peripheral nerves. It plays an important role in managing vital functions such as heart rate, breathing, sleeping, and eating. It regulates the central nervous system and is pivotal in maintaining consciousness and regulating the sleep cycle.

Broca's area: An area in the frontal lobe of the dominant hemisphere (the left one, for most people) near the base of the motor cortex. It produces speech, interprets hand gestures and the actions of others, and assists working memory.

central nervous system: The majority of the nervous system, located within the skull and spine and consisting of the brain and spinal cord. It integrates information it receives from all parts of the body and coordinates and influences the activity of these parts as well.

cerebellum: (Latin for "little brain") A large structure at the back of the brain (below the occipital lobe), which plays an important role in motor control, posture, and balance. It does not initiate movement, but it fine-tunes motor activity for coordination, precision, and accurate timing.

cerebral cortex: The uppermost, folded outer layer of the brain, which is divided into two halves, or hemispheres.

cerebrum: (Latin for "brain") A structure that includes the cerebral cortex as well as several subcortical structures, including the hippocampus, basal ganglia, and olfactory bulb.

circadian rhythms: Physical, mental, and behavioral changes that follow a roughly 24-hour cycle, responding primarily to light and darkness in the environment. They are found in most living things, including animals, plants, and microbes. The study of circadian rhythms is called chronobiology.

cognitive neuroscience: An academic field concerned with the scientific study of the biological substrates underlying cognition, and how psychological functions and behavior are produced by neural circuits in the brain.

cortisol: A steroid hormone produced in the adrenal gland in response to stress and low blood glucose. It increases blood flow and blood sugar; suppresses the immune system; aids in the metabolism of fat, protein, and carbohydrates; and decreases bone formation. Cortisol affects most cells in the body.

dendrite: A branched, treelike structure attached to the cell body of a neuron that receives incoming information from other neurons across the synapse and sends the information into the neuron for further processing. It is part of the brain's gray matter.

dopamine: A major neurotransmitter that plays a significant role in addiction, alertness, attention, learning, voluntary movement, the perception of pain and pleasure, and reward-linked behavior, including addiction. Parkinson's disease is characterized by the gradual death of dopamine-producing neurons.

entropy (adj., entropic): The degree of disorder or uncertainty in a system; a process of degradation.

executive functions: A set of abilities that direct nonroutinized behavior for self-determined goals. Executive functions include working memory, reasoning, task flexibility, and problem solving, as well as planning and execution. They provide verbal access to mental states for self-talk and emotional regulation.

GABA (gamma-aminobutyric acid): The chief inhibitory neurotransmitter, which plays the leading role in reducing neuronal excitability throughout the nervous system. It also regulates muscle tone in humans.

generative (n., generativity): Having the power or function of originating, producing, or reproducing.

glia: Nonneural support cells of the nervous system that perform important housekeeping functions, such as supplying neurons with resources, removing waste, and protecting neurons from toxins and threats. They also influence the transmission of information between neurons.

glutamate: An amino acid, the major excitatory and most prevalent neurotransmitter. Glutamate is involved in most aspects of normal brain function, including cognition, learning, memory, movement, perception, neuroplasticity, and the pruning of connections, as well as metabolism and the survival of neurons.

gray matter: Areas of the brain made up of neuronal cell bodies, *dendrites*, and synapses.

gut bacteria: Also known as gut flora or gut microbiota, a complex community of microorganism species that live in the digestive tracts of animals. Gut bacteria perform many important digestive functions and mediate immune system activity. The average person has about 100 trillion microorganisms in the intestines—ten times the number of human cells in the body.

hippocampus: A cortical seahorse-shaped structure that lies deep inside the temporal lobe and is part of the limbic system and the default network brain asset. The hippocampus orchestrates memory functions, such as storing new information in long-term memory, memory retrieval, and working memory. It also plays an important role in spatial navigation, dreaming, and identity. This structure is compromised in the early stages of Alzheimer's disease.

homeostasis: A self-regulating process by which an organism maintains inner stability while adjusting to external conditions. The stability attained is a dynamic equilibrium, in which continuous change occurs, yet relatively uniform conditions prevail. In humans, the goals of homeostasis include facilitating movement, energy procurement, maintenance of the body's integrity, ensuring species continuation, and social regulation. If homeostasis is successful, life continues; if it fails, disaster or death ensues.

hypothalamus: A collection of small limbic structures just above the brain stem that integrate autonomic functions within the brain and link the nervous system to the endocrine system via the pituitary gland. It provides important functions related to homeostasis, body temperature, hunger, thirst, fatigue, sleep, circadian rhythms, and species-typical parenting and attachment behaviors.

identity: The distinguishing character or personality of an individual; individuality.

inflammation: The body's immunovascular response to harmful stimuli, such as pathogens, damaged cells, or irritants. The purpose of inflammation is to eliminate the cause of cell injury, to clear out dead cells and tissues damaged by the inflammatory process, and to initiate tissue repair. It can be acute or chronic.

insula: A limbic structure embedded deep within the temporal lobe, linked to important activity including consciousness, emotion (especially disgust), homeostasis, interpersonal experience, and motor control.

limbic system: A set of subcortical brain structures linked to emotion, memory, mood, rewards, social activity, stress, and homeostasis.

melatonin: A hormone secreted at night by the pineal gland that plays a role in circadian and seasonal rhythms.

memory: The power of mind to recall at will what has been learned and retained, especially through associative mechanisms.

mental range of motion: The main parameters of human mental activity produced by the five key brain assets discussed in this book: achievement, adaptation, adventure, attachment, and autobiography.

mind: The part of a person that thinks, reasons, feels, and remembers.

motivation: The condition of being eager to act or work. Extrinsic motivation arises from factors outside an individual, such as duty, money, fame, grades, praise, or social recognition. Intrinsic motivation is triggered by factors within the person, such as enjoyment, integrity, meaning, or a sense of satisfaction.

myelin: An insulating material that surrounds axons to enhance electrical conduction. Myelinated axons are capable of carrying messages at almost three hundred miles per hour. Myelin, composed mainly of water and lipids (particularly cholesterol), has a whitish color and is referred to as the brain's white matter.

narrative: A story: an account of related events, actual or imaginary, with a beginning, middle, and end, presented in a sequence of words (written or spoken), images (still or moving), sounds (music), physical movements (facial expressions, hand gestures, or whole-body movements), or objects, or by other means.

nerves: Bands of fibers that transmit information between the brain, muscles, spinal cord, and organs of the body. Nerves are composed of axons, dendrites, and protective and supportive structures.

nervous system: The communication network that connects the brain and the body's cells and structures. The two main branches of the nervous system in humans (and all vertebrates) are the central nervous system (within the skull and spine) and the peripheral nervous system (outside the skull and spine).

neurogenesis: The development of new neurons or nervous tissue.

neuron: A cell that communicates with other cells via electrochemical messages sent through nerves. The neuron is the basic functional unit of the nervous system.

neuroplasticity: Changes in brain anatomy, chemistry, and physiology due to changes in relationships, experiences, behavior, environment, experience, health, thinking, emotions, bodily injury, and other factors.

neurosis: An emotional disorder in which a person experiences strong feelings of fear or worry. The condition affects only part of the personality, is accompanied by a less-distorted perception of reality than in a psychosis, does not impair the use of language, and is accompanied by various physical, physiological, and mental disturbances (such as visceral symptoms, anxieties, or phobias).

neurotransmitter: A chemical generated within the body that transmits signals across a synapse from one neuron to another. A neurotransmitter can excite or inhibit a neuron's response. Over one hundred neurotransmitters influence the brain; about thirty of these are also found in the gut brain (neurons within the gastrointestinal tract). Most of the brain's work is conducted by the major neurotransmitters acetylcholine, dopamine, GABA, glutamate, melatonin, norepinephrine, and serotonin.

norepinephrine: Also called noradrenaline, a stress hormone and excitatory neurotransmitter that is synthesized from its close chemical neighbor, dopamine. Norepinephrine has widespread influence throughout the brain. It mediates behavioral and physiological responses to unpleasant stimuli, and it is associated with vigilant concentration and readiness to act in response to a stimulus.

oxytocin: A major social hormone and neurotransmitter produced by the hypothalamus. Oxytocin plays a role in trust, intimacy, pair bonding, sexual reproduction of both sexes, childbirth, lactation, and parental activity. It decreases the influence of cortisol and boosts immune activity. It relieves fear, anxiety, and pain in the presence of social support.

peripheral nervous system: The part of the nervous system that lies mainly outside the skull and spine. It includes the cranial nerves and the spinal nerves. The two main components of the peripheral nervous system are the *autonomic nervous system* (which manages internal conditions of homeostasis) and the somatic nervous system (which sends and receives information to the brain pertaining to the external environment and motor activity).

personality: The emotional and behavioral characteristics that distinguish one person from another.

rational (n., rationality): Based on facts or reason rather than feelings; capable of reasoning or thinking clearly about things.

resilience: The ability to bounce back and return to inner equilibrium (homeostasis) after an adverse event.

serotonin: A feel-good neurotransmitter connected to social activity and sunlight that influences appetite, learning, memory, mood, sensory perception, and sleep.

soul: The whole-person blueprint in each person that is built out through the individual's life story.

spirit: Awareness of the invisible life force within and around the self.

synapse: The physical space where one neuron connects with another by sending and receiving chemically encoded messages.

synaptic connection: A working relationship between two neurons at a synapse.

telomere: The protective cap at the end of a chromosome that protects genetic information from deterioration and influences health and aging outcomes.

thalamus: An egg-shaped mass of neurons in each hemisphere at the center of the brain that relays sensory information to and from the cerebral cortex.

theory of mind: A set of abilities for understanding the mental states—the beliefs, desires, feelings, intentions, motivations, and perspectives—of other people, and for realizing how their mental states are different from our own. A theory of mind enables the development of narratives to understand and predict the behavior of oneself and others.

vagus nerve: The tenth cranial nerve. It provides a link between the central nervous system and the body for parasympathetic control of the heart, lungs, and digestive tract.

vasopressin: A major social hormone and neurotransmitter produced by the hypothalamus. Its primary functions are to retain water in the body and to constrict blood vessels. Vasopressin plays a key role in homeostasis through regulation of water, glucose, and salts in the blood. It influences pair bonding, parental activity, and social behavior.

Wernicke's area: A region of the brain that enables the comprehension of language, located in the temporal lobe near the junction with the parietal lobe. In most people, it is located in the left hemisphere.

working memory: A mental scratch pad that allows manipulation of new information in conjunction with information stored in memory to facilitate learning, problem solving, and the generation of ideas.

Resources by chapter

Introduction

If this painfully brief overview of neurons and neuroplasticity whets your appetite to learn more about neuroanatomy, I suggest you consult Rita Carter's *The Human Brain Book* (listed below under Publications). Her book *Mapping the Mind* was the first book I ever read about the brain, almost fifteen years ago, and obviously it hooked me. For a book that takes a mind-body-spirit view of the brain, I suggest Adam Zeman's *A Portrait of the Brain* (listed below under Publications).

Chapter 1: What Success Looks Like

To learn more about brain hype, see Leon Eisenberg's "Were we all asleep at the switch? A personal reminiscence of psychiatry from 1940 to 2010" (listed below under Research).

For insider information about the limits of neuroscience findings, read Robert Burton's book *A Skeptic's Guide to the Mind* (listed below under Publications).

Early in the twentieth century, Picasso studied primitive art, fascinated by the powerful emotional impact it conveyed. This primary focus on emotions presaged the neuroscientific revolution on emotions described in Antonio Damasio's book *Descartes' Error* (listed below under Publications) by almost one hundred years.

Chapter 2: A Brain for All Ages

If you are interested in learning more about the human body's evolutionary history, check out Neil Shubin's *Your Inner Fish* (listed below under Publications), which was also the theme of a PBS special program. For an in-depth look at how the head and brain coevolved, consult Daniel

Lieberman's *The Evolution of the Human Head* (listed below under Publications). To learn more about the deep underpinnings of human social behavior, read primatologist Frans de Waal's classic work *Chimpanzee Politics* (listed below under Publications), which is required reading for newly elected Congressional representatives.

Chapter 3: Brain Assets

If you would like to learn more detail about Brodmann's areas and functions attributed to specific areas, the Sylvius 4 Online resource (listed below under Websites) is worth the annual subscription of $25. The Carlson textbook *Physiology of Behavior* (listed below under Publications) is more expensive and technical, as well as more informative, about brain areas.

Chapter 4: The Brain Portfolio Tool

While in-person classes are best for brain asset optimization, I believe there is a place for online learning too. An online course in a subject that interests you may be effective. Just avoid spending too much time in front of a screen.

Chapter 6: Honing the Superpowers

For a compelling look at our superpowers in action that is also a quick read, try Viktor Frankl's *Man's Search for Meaning* or C. S. Lewis' *The Abolition of Man.* If you'd like a deeper look at the emotional aspects of the human condition, read Carl Jung's *Modern Man in Search of a Soul,* which includes a description of the original research underlying the theories that led to the Myers-Briggs personality type system. For an interesting perspective on job-related stress, see Arlie Hochschild's *The Managed Heart.* (All four books are listed below under Publications.)

Chapter 7: The Better with Age Lifestyle

For more information about neuroscientists' views on brain training, see "A Consensus on the Brain Training Industry from the Scientific Community" (listed below under Websites).

For more information about the SuperAging Study, see the website for "Cognitive Neurology and Alzheimer's Disease Center" (listed below under Websites).

For a searing artistic perspective on what causes Alzheimer's, see Tony Kushner's work *The Intelligent Homosexual's Guide* (listed below under Publications).

For helpful insights about the role of fats in brain and body health, see Susan Allport's *The Queen of Fats* (listed below under Publications).

If you are interested in maintaining a healthy mind-body-spirit lifestyle wherever you live, I highly recommend learning more about Ayurveda, starting with Vasant Lad's book (listed below under Publications).

The principles of Ayurveda (a Sanskrit term translated as "life knowledge" or "the science of self-healing") originated thousands of years ago and were organized and incorporated into the Vedic scriptures of Hinduism some three thousand years ago. The Ayurvedic tradition is based on a deep understanding of nature and culture as a context for human mind-body-spirit health. Ayurvedic techniques are still used in many Indian hospitals today.

One of the most useful concepts in Ayurveda is a focus on the gastrointestinal tract as the foundation of mind-body-spirit health. Ayurveda uses food as medicine and employs fasting, herbal remedies, massage, meditation, minerals, yoga, and other lifestyle interventions to heal the physical damage that toxic emotions can inflict on the body. The mind is guided toward health-promoting activity and away from self-destructive activity.

The religious beliefs that brought meaning and social cohesion to people living in the Indus Valley three thousand years ago do not resonate with me, but their integrative health techniques work anyway. You can use the techniques without subscribing to the worldview that birthed them. Find what works for you, and don't drink the Kool-Aid.

Additional Resources

Publications

Allport, Susan. *The Queen of Fats: Why Omega-3s Were Removed from the Western Diet and What We Can Do to Replace Them.* Berkeley: University of California Press, 2008.

Burton, Robert. *A Skeptic's Guide to the Mind: What Neuroscience Can and Cannot Tell Us about Ourselves.* New York: St. Martin's Press, 2013.

Byrnes, James. *Minds, Brains, and Learning: Understanding the Psychological and Educational Relevance of Neuroscientific Research.* New York: Guilford Press, 2001.

Carlson, Neil. *Physiology of Behavior.* 11th ed. New York: Pearson Education, Inc., 2012.

Carstensen, Laura. *A Long Bright Future: Happiness, Health, and Financial Security in an Age of Increased Longevity.* New York: PublicAffairs, 2011.

Carter, Rita. *The Human Brain Book.* London: Dorling Kindersley, 2014.

Cozolino, Louis. *The Healthy Aging Brain: Sustaining Attachment, Attaining Wisdom.* New York: Norton, 2008.

Damasio, Antonio. *Descartes' Error: Emotion, Reason and the Human Brain.* New York: Penguin Group, 1994.

———. *Self Comes to Mind: Constructing the Conscious Brain.* New York: Vintage Books, 2012.

De Waal, Frans. *Chimpanzee Politics: Power and Sex among the Apes.* Baltimore: The Johns Hopkins University Press, 1998.

Einstein, Albert. *The Expanded Quotable Einstein.* 2nd ed. Edited by Alice Calaprice. Princeton: Princeton University Press, 2000.

Frankl, Viktor. *Man's Search for Meaning.* Boston: Beacon Press, 2006.

Hochschild, Arlie Russell. *The Managed Heart: The Commercialization of Human Feeling.* Berkeley: University of California Press, 2012.

James, William. *The Varieties of Religious Experience: A Study In Human Nature.* New York: Simon and Schuster, 1997.

Jung, Carl. *Modern Man in Search of a Soul.* San Diego: Harcourt Harvest, 1955.

———. *Man and His Symbols.* New York: Dell Publishing, 1968.

Kotre, John. *Outliving the Self: Generativity and the Interpretation of Lives.* Baltimore: The Johns Hopkins University Press, 1984.

Kushner, Tony. *The Intelligent Homosexual's Guide to Capitalism and Socialism with a Key to the Scriptures.* New York: Theatre Communications Group, 2009.

Lad, Vasant. *Ayurveda: The Science of Self-Healing.* Twin Lakes, WI: Lotus Press, 1985.

LeDoux, Joseph. *The Emotional Brain: The Mysterious Underpinnings of Emotional Life.* New York: Simon and Schuster, 1998.

———. *Synaptic Self: How Our Brains Become Who We Are.* New York: Penguin Group, 2003.

Lewis, C. S. *The Abolition of Man.* New York: HarperOne, 2015.

Lieberman, Daniel. *The Evolution of the Human Head.* Cambridge: Harvard University Press, 2011.

Sedlar, Jeri, and Miners, Rick. *Don't Retire, Rewire!* 2nd ed. New York: Alpha Books, 2007.

Shubin, Neil. *Your Inner Fish: A Journey into the 3.5-Billion-Year History of the Human Body*. New York: Vintage Books, 2009.

Snowdon, David. *Aging with Grace: What the Nun Study Teaches Us about Leading Longer, Healthier, and More Meaningful Lives*. New York: Bantam Books, 2002.

Vaillant, George. *Aging Well: Surprising Guideposts to a Happier Life from the Landmark Harvard Study of Adult Development*. New York: Little Brown, 2003.

———. *Spiritual Evolution: How We Are Wired for Faith, Hope, and Love*. New York: Harmony Books, 2009.

Zeman, Adam. *A Portrait of the Brain*. New Haven: Yale University Press, 2008.

Research Articles and Studies

Andrews-Hanna, J. L., J. Smallwood, and R. N. Spreng. "The default network and self-generated thought: Component processes, dynamic control, and clinical relevance." *Annals of the New York Academy of Sciences* 1316 (May 2014): 29–52. doi:10.1111/nyas.12360.

Buckner, R. L., J. L. Andrews-Hanna, and D. L. Schachter. "The brain's default network: Anatomy, function, and relevance to disease." *Annals of the New York Academy of Sciences* 1124 (March 2008): 1–38. doi:10.1196/annals.1440.011.

Eisenberg, L., and L. B. Guttmacher. "Were we all asleep at the switch? A personal reminiscence of psychiatry from 1940 to 2010." *Acta Psychiatrica Scandinavica* 122: 89–102. doi: 10.1111/j.1600-0447.2010.01544.x (2010). http://onlinelibrary.wiley.com/doi/10.1111/j.1600-0447.2010.01544.x/full.

Etkin, A., T. Egner, and R. Kalisch. "Emotional processing in anterior cingulate and medial prefrontal cortex." *Trends in Cognitive Sciences* 15(2) (February 2011): 85–93.

Institute of Medicine. *Cognitive Aging: Progress in Understanding and Opportunities for Action*. Washington, DC: National Academies Press, 2015. http://books.nap.edu/openbook.php?record_id=21693.

National Research Council and Institute of Medicine. *U.S. Health in International Perspective: Shorter Lives, Poorer Health*. Washington, DC: National Academies Press, 2013. http://books.nap.edu/openbook.php?record_id=13497.

Royal Society, UK. Brain Waves. Ongoing project investigating developments in neuroscience and their implications for society and public policy. https://royalsociety.org/policy/projects/brain-waves/.

Websites

A Consensus on the Brain Training Industry from the Scientific Community. A letter published jointly by the Stanford Center on Longevity and the Max

Planck Institute for Human Development objecting to claims made by the brain training industry. http://longevity3.stanford.edu/blog/2014/10/15 /the-consensus-on-the-brain-training-industry-from-the-scientific-community-2/.

American Psychological Association. Tips for building resilience. http://www .apa.org/helpcenter/road-resilience.aspx#, accessed July 3, 2015.

Brain Facts, Society for Neuroscience. Basic information and educational resources about the brain. www.brainfacts.org.

Brain Wealth: Programs offered by Phyllis Strupp, author of *Better with Age*. Video on brain training and signup for free monthly e-tip are available: http://www.brainwealth.org.

Center for Brain Health, University of Texas. Free daily update about brain research findings from around the world. www.brainhealthdaily.com.

Cognitive Neurology and Alzheimer's Disease Center, Northwestern University. Resources and information on the SuperAging Study. http://brain .northwestern.edu/research/studies/sa.html.

EdX. Website offering MOOCs (massive open online courses) from many major universities for free. Some offer certificates of completion. www.edx .org.

Khan Academy. Free online, self-paced classes on topics such as math, art, computer programming, economics, physics, chemistry, biology, medicine, finance, and history. www.khanacademy.org.

Neuroscience for Kids. Basic information and educational resources about the brain geared toward kids but helpful for adults. Free monthly newsletter shares information about websites and recent media coverage about the brain. http://faculty.washington.edu/chudler/neurok.html.

Project Neuron, University of Illinois. Novel educational materials for understanding research on neuroscience. Middle- and high-school science curriculum materials that emphasize inquiry and active learning. http:// neuron.illinois.edu.

Science Update Spotlight: The Brain, American Association of Arts and Sciences. Collection of sixty-second podcasts about new discoveries in science, technology, and medicine. www.scienceupdate.com/spotlights /the-brain/.

Sylvius 4 Online: An Interactive Atlas and Visual Glossary of Human Neuroanatomy, Sinauer Associates. http://sylvius.sinauer.com.

World Health Rankings. Rate of Alzheimer's/dementia deaths by country. www.worldlifeexpectancy.com/cause-of-death/alzheimers-dementia/ by-country, accessed July 3, 2015.

"Your Brain" exhibit, Franklin Institute. www.fi.edu/exhibit/your-brain.

FIGURE CREDITS

International Perspective, listed in the Resources section under Research Articles and Studies.

page 123: Average life expectancy data is from the National Research Council's study *U.S. Health in International Perspective*. Rate of Alzheimer's/dementia deaths by country is from the World Health Organization, accessed at www.worldlifeexpectancy.com /cause-of-death/alzheimers-dementia/by-country on July 3, 2015.

page 128: Megan Cott, stickfigureeconomics.blogspot.com

page 129: Jason Love, cartoonstock.com

page 133: Endrio Amoroso, Crevision, www.crevision.dk

INDEX

Page numbers followed by *f* indicate figures. Page numbers in **bold** indicate definitions in the glossary.

exercise of. *See* physical exercise movement of. *See* physical movement

brain, 21–37. *See also specific functions and parts of brain*
  changes with age to, 1, 14, 21, 63, 113
  complexity of, 2, 102, 113
  development of, 30–37, 31f, 127
  evolution of, 22–30, 25f
  injuries to, recovery from, 3–4
  integration of areas of. *See* integration
  life story approach to, 22
  vs. mind, 46
  myths about, 21
  resource consumption by, 23, 26
  size of, 2, 23, 26
  as social organ, xvi
  structure of, 24, 25f, 40–43, 41f, 42f
  warranty conditions for, 2, 76

brain assets, 39–58. *See also* default network; frontal lobe; occipital lobe; parietal lobe; temporal lobe
  activities for engaging, 68f–69f, 70–73
  attributes of, 64–65, 66f
  defining, 40–43
  development of concept, xvi
  difficulty of measuring, 76
  evidence of growth in, 75–76
  growth of, as goal of brain training, 63–64
  identifying underperforming, 60–62, 65–70
  introduction of five, 41–42
  management of. *See* Brain Portfolio Tool
  mental dimensions of. *See* mental range of motion
  qualities, quips, and analogues associated with, 48–57
  relative efficiency of, 70
  returns on investment in, 65, 67f
  self-assessment of, 71–73, 74f

tips for growing, 75–87
brain buddies, 86
BRAIN Initiative, 115
brain portfolio
  development of concept, 39–40
  need for diversification of, 63
  value of, 62–64
Brain Portfolio Tool, 59–73
  brain asset activities in, 68f–69f, 70–71
  brain asset attributes in, 64–65, 66f
  brain asset returns in, 65, 67f
  definition of, 17
  development of concept, xvi, 59–62
  engaging underperforming assets in, 60–62, 65–70
  increase in brain wealth as goal of, 63–64
  overview of, 64–71
  self-assessment of assets in, 71–73, 74f
brain stem, **136**
  development of, 31
  evolution of, 24–26, 25f
  functions of, 40, 136
  location of, 40, 41f
brain training
  definition of, ix, 4–6
  frequently asked questions about, ix–x
  increase in brain wealth as goal of, 63–64
  meaning of success in, 9, 13–20
  physical training compared to, 4–5
brain wealth. *See* brain assets
Brideshead Revisited (Waugh), 131
Broca's area, 43f, **136**
Brodmann, Korbinian, 41–42
Brodmann areas, 41–42, 43f

caffeine, 102–3
Campbell, Joseph, 113
cannabis, 102–3
carbohydrates, 103

cave drawings, 28f
Cave of the Hands, 28f
central nervous system, 23, **136**. *See also*
   brain
cerebellum, **136-37**
   development of, 31
   evolution of, 24, 25f
   functions of, 40, 136-37
   location of, 40, 41f
cerebral cortex, **137**. *See also* frontal
   lobe; occipital lobe; parietal lobe;
   temporal lobe
   brain assets in, 40-45
   Brodmann areas of, 41-42, 43f
   development of, 31, 35
cerebrum, 25f, 42f, **137**
chemical substances, neurotransmitters
   affected by, 102-3
chess, 78-79
children
   brain development in, 31, 32-34
   judgments about capabilities of, 104
   tips for growing brain assets of, 77-79
chronobiology, 137
Churchill, Winston, 129
cingulate cortex. *See also* anterior
      cingulate cortex
   in limbic system, 41
   posterior, 93, 93f, 95
   regions of, 93, 93f
   in superpowers, 93, 93f
circadian rhythms, **137**
Cloud of Unknowing, The, 105
cocaine, 103
cognitive control network
   development of, 30, 31f, 33-34, 92
   superpowers supported by, 92
cognitive flexibility, importance of, 71,
   95
Cognitive Neurology and Alzheimer's
   Disease Center, 117-18
cognitive neuroscience, 46, **137**. *See also*
   scientific research

collective brain wealth, of humans, 63
communication
   between hemispheres of brain, 42-45,
      71, 81
   by neurons, 1, 2f
compound interest, 63
computer-based brain training games,
   116
consciousness, regulation of, 24-26
corpus callosum, 42f, 44
cortisol, 6-7, **137**
cranial nerves, 25f
cultural tools, supported by brain assets,
   65, 67f
culture
   in Alzheimer's disease, 115, 123-25
   Italian, 119-21
   and Super-Agers, 121-25
   value of brain assets in U.S., 128-29

Darwin, Charles, *The Descent of Man,* 10
default network
   activities for engaging, 69f, 70-71
   in Alzheimer's disease, 115
   attributes of, 64-65, 66f
   autobiography associated with, 56,
      66f, 75, 101
   development of, 30, 31f, 33-35, 92, 127
   evolution of, 25f
   introduction as brain asset, 42
   as less efficient asset, 70
   qualities, quips, and analogues
      associated with, 56-57
   returns on investment in, 65, 67f
   superpowers supported by, 92-93
   tips for growing, 84
dementia
   brain assets affected by, 32
   international comparison of rates of,
      123-25, 123f
   presenile, 114. *See also* Alzheimer's
      disease
   senile, 114

HPA axis. *See* hypothalamus-
pituitary-adrenal axis
human brain. *See* brain
Human Brain Project, 115
Human Connectome Project, 115
hypothalamus, **139**
  evolution of, 24–26
  functions of, 6–7, 41, 139
  in limbic system, 41, 42f
  in stress response system, 6–7, 41
hypothalamus-pituitary-adrenal (HPA)
  axis, 6–7

Iceland, Alzheimer's disease in, 125
identity, **139**
  alignment of goals with, 84
  autobiographical self, 26, 36–37, 84
  challenges of changing, 89
  whole-person, 46–47
immune system, effects of stress on, 7–8
Indonesia, Mount Koba in, 26–27
inflammation, **139**
  effects of stress on, 7–8
injuries, brain, recovery from, 3–4
inner movements, 7, 76. *See also*
  emotion
Institute of Medicine, 121
insula, 41, 94, **139**
integration of brain
  brain assets in, 47, 70
  in development of brain, 31, 31f, 35, 127
  as product of aging, 14, 63
  scientific research on, 24–26, 59
intelligence quotient (IQ), 21
intentions
  in learning, 75
  of others, in theory of mind, 90, 107f,
  143
interest, compound, 63
intrinsic motivation, 84, 97, 140
investment in brain assets,, returns on,
  65, 67f
Invictus (Henley), 73

IQ (intelligence quotient), 21
Italy
  Alzheimer's disease in, 121, 123f, 124
  life expectancy in, 121, 122f
  lifestyle of, 119–21
  Super-Agers in, 121, 124

James, William, 126
Japan, 124f
  Alzheimer's disease in, 123f, 124
  life expectancy in, 121, 122f, 123f, 124
  Super-Agers in, 124
Jung, Carl, 39, 126

Keller, Helen, 64
Kierkegaard, Søren, 89
Koba, Mount, 26–27

language
  in development of brain, 31, 33
  frontal lobe in, 71
  verbal access to mental states, 9, 110f,
  138
leadership, brain-asset, 70
learning
  anxiety in, 79, 80
  brain asset growth through, 73
  as evidence of growth in brain wealth,
  75, 76
  as key to neuroplasticity, 4
  need for lifelong, 76
  social context for, 73, 79, 100, 104
  working memory in, 95
Leaves of Grass (Whitman), 132, 133
left hemisphere of brain
  bilateral specialization of, 24, 42
  brain assets in, 42–43
  communication with right hemisphere, 42–45, 71, 81
  development of, 31
  functions of, 42–43, 44f
life expectancy
  by country, 121–25, 122f, 123f

life expectancy (*continued*)
  living long vs. living well, 17–19,
    123–25
life story approach to brain, 22
lifestyle, 113–31
  and Alzheimer's disease, 114–16, 123–25
  changes since World War II to, 127–29
  and health in U.S. vs. other countries,
    121–25
  of Italians, 119–21
  of Super-Agers, 9, 116–19, 125–26
life-work balance struggle, 34, 83
limbic system, **140**
  components of, 41, 42f, 93
  evolution of, 24, 25f
  functions of, 41
Lincoln, Abraham, 86
LSD, 103

Maclean, Paul, 24
mammals, evolution of brain of, 25f
Marcus Aurelius, 10
marijuana, 102–3
MDMA, 103
media coverage, of Alzheimer's
  disease, 13
melatonin, **140**
  evolution of, 23, 24
  production of, 24
memory, **140**
  changes with age to, 14, 21, 35
  in development of brain, 35, 36
  and difficulty of measuring brain
    assets, 76
  mind as, 46
  parts of brain responsible for, 40, 41,
    42
  working. *See* working memory
men, life expectancies of, 121
mental range of motion, 4–6, **140**. *See
  also* achievement; adaptation;
  adventure; attachment;
  autobiography

  importance of using full, 4, 47, 101,
    128–29
  introduction of five dimensions of, 5
mental states
  of others, in theory of mind, 33, 90,
    107f, 143
  verbal access to, 9, 110f, 138
mid-cingulate, 93, 93f
midlife crises, 35
Millennial Generation, 79–81
mind. *See also* memory
  vs. brain, 46
  definition of, 46, **140**
  exercise of, 5–6
  group or hive, 100
  as memory, 46
  in stages of brain development, 34
  theory of. *See* theory of mind
  use of term, 46
mind-body-spirit health, xv
Mitchell, Joni, 91
mojo, 89–90
money
  neurotransmitters affected by, 103
  pursuit of, xiii–xv
morphine, 103
Moses, Grandma, 116–17, 116f
motivations, **140**
  extrinsic, 84, **140**
  intrinsic, 84, 97, **140**
  of others, in theory of mind, 90,
    143
motor output. *See* physical movement
Mount Fuji, 124f
Mount Koba, 26–27
movement(s)
  of body. *See* physical movement
  emotion as source of, 6
  inner, 7, 76. *See also* emotion
multigenerational living, 127
music, origins of, xii–xiii
myelin, 33, **140**
myths, about brain, 21

narratives, **140**
  in Story Superpower, 91, 107f, 110f–11f
  in theory of mind, 90, 143
National Research Council, 121
neocortex, 24, 25f
neomammalian complex of brain, 24
nerve(s), **140**
  cranial, 25f
  evolution of, 23, 25f
  vagus, 7, 8f, **143**
nervous system, **140–41**. *See also* brain
  autonomic, **135–36**
  central, 23, **136**
  evolution of, 23
  peripheral, **142**
neurofibrillary tangles, 114
neurogenesis, 33, **141**
neurons, **141**
  in brain portfolio, 63
  communication by, 1, 2f
  connections between. *See* synaptic
    connections
  in development of brain, 32–33
  evolution of, 23
  functions of, 1–2
  number of, 2, 63
  origins of term, 23
  spindle, 25f, 93–94, 94f
  structure of, 1
neuroplasticity, **141**. *See also* brain
    assets; brain training
  improvements with age in, 1, 113
  learning as key to, 4
  need for, 76
  in recovery from brain injuries, 3–4
  resilience in, 9
  value of, 63
neuroscience, cognitive, 46, **137**. *See also*
    scientific research
neurosis, 2, **141**
neurotransmitters, **141**. *See also specific*
    types
  evolution of, 23, 29

functions of, 23
substances affecting, 102–3
types of, 23
nicotine, 103
nonroutinized behavior, executive
  functions directing, 34, 90, 108f–9f,
  138
noradrenaline. *See* norepinephrine
norepinephrine, **141**
  functions of, 141
  and inflammation, 7
  substances affecting release of, 103
Northwestern University, 117–18, 125
nuns, research on brains of, 114, 126

occipital lobe
  achievement associated with, 50, 66f,
    75, 101
  activities for engaging, 68f, 70–71
  attributes of, 64–65, 66f
  Brodmann areas for, 41, 43f
  development of, 31–32
  introduction as brain asset, 41–42
  as more efficient asset, 70
  qualities, quips, and analogues associ-
    ated with, 50–51
  returns on investment in, 65, 67f
opiates, 103
oxytocin, **141–42**
  evolution of, 29
  functions of, 141–42
  and learning, 73, 100, 104

paleomammalian complex of brain, 24
parasympathetic nervous system, 136
parietal lobe
  activities for engaging, 68f, 70–71,
    97–102
  adventure associated with, 48, 66f, 75,
    101
  attributes of, 64–65, 66f
  Brodmann areas for, 41, 43f
  development of, 31–32

parietal lobe (*continued*)
  introduction as brain asset, 41
  as more efficient asset, 70
  qualities, quips, and analogues associated with, 48–49
  returns on investment in, 65, 67f
  tips for growing, 80, 82
  as underperforming asset, 60
  in working memory, 80, 95, 97–102
Parkinson's disease, 41, 91, 137
PCC. *See* posterior cingulate cortex
peripheral nervous system, **142**
personality, **142**
  and superpowers, 104
perspective(s)
  mind-body-spirit, xv
  of others, in theory of mind, 90, 107f, 143
  whole-person, 46–47
physical exercise, 4–6
  brain training compared to, 4–5
  in growth of brain assets, 80–81, 82
  and working memory, 80, 100–102
physical fitness, major dimensions of, 5
physical movement (motor output)
  in activities to engage brain assets, 68f–69f, 70–71
  communication between hemispheres in, 42–43, 71, 81
  evolution of, 22
  forms of, 71
  parts of brain responsible for, 40–43, 71, 81
Picasso, Jacqueline, 18
Picasso, Pablo, 17–19, 18f, 75, 79
pineal gland, 24, 25f
pituitary gland
  in limbic system, 41
  in stress response system, 6–7, 41
plaques, amyloid
  in Alzheimer's disease, 114, 115f
  in Super-Agers, 118
Porter, Cole, 16

portfolio, brain. *See* brain portfolio
Portugal, Alzheimer's disease in, 123f, 124
posterior cingulate cortex (PCC), 93, 93f, 95
prefrontal cortex, 95
presenile dementia, 114. *See also* Alzheimer's disease
puberty, development of brain in, 33–34

quips, associated with brain assets, 49, 51, 53, 55, 57

racial stereotypes, and superpowers, 104
Ramón y Cajal, Santiago, 13, 47
Raphael, 119
rationality, **142**
  in development of brain, 31
  evolution of, 29
  myths about, 21
  in Super-Agers, 118–19
  in superpowers, 91, 95
reading, 105
Reagan, Nancy, 18f
Reagan, Ronald, 17–18, 18f
reasoning. *See* rationality
relationships. *See also* social connections
  importance of, xiv, xvi, 126
  in resilience, 126
  in Self Superpower, 91, 106f
  sensory-motor functions in experience of, 90, 91, 106f
relaxation response, vagus nerve in, 7
reptiles, evolution of brain of, 25f
reptilian complex of brain, 24
research. *See* scientific research
resilience
  approaches to increasing, 126
  definition of, 9, **142**
  of Super-Agers, 9, 125–26
resource consumption, by brain, 23, 26

retirement
as "rewirement," 17
tips for growing brain assets in,
84-86
returns on investment, in brain assets,
65, 67f
Richest of Fare, The (Strupp), xiv, 59, 126
right hemisphere of brain
bilateral specialization of, 24, 42
brain assets in, 42-43
communication with left hemisphere,
42-45
communication with right hemisphere, 71, 81
development of, 31
functions of, 42-43, 44f
Rolling Stone (magazine), 35-36
Roosevelt, Eleanor, 37
rumination, 125

scientific research
on Alzheimer's disease, 13-14, 114-16
on development of brain, 30
on health in U.S. vs. other countries,
121-25
on integration of brain, 24-26, 59
on neuroplasticity, 113
on structure of brain, 24-26
on Super-Agers, 117-18, 125
self, autobiographical, 26, 36-37, 84
self-assessment
of brain assets, 71-73, 74f
of superpowers, 102-5, 106f-9f
self-consciousness, 26
self-determined goals, executive functions in, 34, 90, 138
self-limiting thoughts and beliefs, 104
self-reliance, xvi
Self Superpower, 91-94, 92f
activities for honing, 104, 110f
self-assessment of, 106f
and Super-Agers, 118
senile dementia, 114

sensory-motor functions (SM), 90-91
definition of, 90
self-assessment of, 106f
as Self Superpower, 91-94, 92f, 106f
sensory-motor network
development of, 30, 31f, 92
superpowers supported by, 92
serotonin, **142**
evolution of, 23, 29
functions of, 142
substances affecting release of, 103
short-term memory. *See* working
memory
Silent Generation, 84-85
sleep, effects of stress on, 7
SM. *See* sensory-motor functions
Snowdon, David, *Aging with Grace*, 114,
126
social connections. *See also*
relationships
evolution of interdependence,
28-30
in learning, 73, 79, 100, 104
need for, 76
social organ, brain as, xvi
social roles, brain development and,
32-36
somatic nervous system, 142
Sondheim, Stephen, 89
soul, 46, **142**
soul force, 92
specialization, bilateral, 24, 42
speech, role of frontal lobe in, 71. *See
also* language
Sperry, Roger, 44
spinal cord, 25f
spindle neurons, 93-94
in animals, 93-94, 94f
evolution of, 25f
functions of, 93
spirit
definition of, 46, **142**
exercise of, 5-6

spirit *(continued)*
in stages of brain development, 35–36
use of term, 46
spontaneity, 22
Star Trek (television show), 18
Steer Superpower, 91–94, 92f
activities for honing, 111f
reliance on input from other super
powers, 104
self-assessment of, 104, 108f–9f
and Super-Agers, 118
and working memory, 95–96
stereotypes, and superpowers, 104
Story Superpower, 91–94, 92f
activities for honing, 110f–11f
self-assessment of, 104, 107f
stress hormones, 6–7. *See also specific
types*
stress management
approaches to, 8–9
in early human history, 28–29
stress response system, 6–9, 8f
substantia nigra, 41
sugar, 103
Sullenberger, Chesley, 95–96, 95f
Sullivan, Annie, 64
Super-Agers, 116–25
anterior cingulate cortex in, 93, 118–19
examples of, 116–17
international distribution of, 123–25
lifestyle of, 9, 116–19, 125–26
resilience of, 9, 125–26
scientific research on, 117–18, 125
secrets of success of, 117–19, 125–26
superpowers, 89–112
activities for honing, 100–102, 104,
110f–11f
anterior cingulate cortex and, 93, 94,
118
in behavior, 94
defining, 90–94
neurological foundation for, 92–94
self-assessment of, 102–5, 106f–9f

in Super-Agers, 118
three types of, 90–91, 91f
working memory and, 94–102
Sweden, Alzheimer's disease in, 123f, 125
Switzerland
Alzheimer's disease in, 123f, 125
life expectancy in, 121, 122f
sympathetic nervous system, 136
synapses, 1, 2f, **142**
synaptic connections, 1–4, **142**
activities for building new, 97–102
after brain injuries, 3–4
challenges of building new, 2–4
in development of brain, 32–33
evidence of new, 75–76
between hemispheres of brain, 44
number of, 2
strength of, 1–2
tips for growing, 77–78

Taylor, Elizabeth, 35–36
telomeres, 8, **142**
temporal lobe
activities for engaging, 68f, 70–71
attachment associated with, 52, 66f,
75, 101
attributes of, 64–65, 66f
Brodmann areas for, 41, 43f
development of, 31–32
introduction as brain asset, 41
as less efficient asset, 70
qualities, quips, and analogues associated with, 52–53
returns on investment in, 65, 67f
tips for growing, 79
thalamus, **143**
evolution of, 24–26
functions of, 40, 143
location of, 40, 41f
THC, 102–3
theory of mind (ToM), 90–91
definition of, 90, **143**
in development of brain, 33